AF254423

this wasn't in the pamphlet

An Unfiltered Guide to Untangling the Mess That Is Type 2 Diabetes

For Real. Promise.

mary van doorn

To everyone who's ever felt ashamed of their diagnosis.
To the ones who've started over more times than they can count.
To those who've had to explain, advocate, educate, and still show up anyway.
You inspired every word of this book.

To the Sugar Mama Strong community and The Sisterhood,
You are the heartbeat behind this mission. You turned a diagnosis into a movement and strangers into family. Your grit, honesty, tears, laughter, and "I'm trying again today" spirit built these pages. Thank you for trusting me with your stories.

And to my family, my constant why, thank you for loving me through every season and believing in me long before I believed in myself.

contents

introduction

(A Note Before We Begin)

When I was first diagnosed with type 2 diabetes, I left the doctor's office with a prescription, a stack of papers, and the vague sense that I should be ashamed of something I barely understood.

The pamphlet told me to lose weight, eat better, and walk more.

It didn't tell me how to handle the fear.

It didn't explain why I suddenly felt like I had to defend my breakfast choices to strangers.

It didn't prepare me for the emotional whiplash of trying to do "everything right" and still seeing numbers that made me feel like a failure.

And it certainly didn't mention the exhaustion of trying so hard and still feeling like it wasn't enough.

This book is for all the things the pamphlet left out.

It's for the in-between moments.

The moments you didn't talk about in the exam room and the ones where you questioned if it was your fault.

The ones where you quietly Googled whether it was too late to "fix" it.

Introduction

The ones where you stared at the medication bottle, wondering what it meant about you.

The ones where you hid how overwhelmed you were because you didn't want to be dramatic, or weak, or "one of those patients."

The ones where you felt like giving up, even though you didn't.

It's also for the quiet wins.

The first time you advocated for yourself.

The day you checked your blood sugar without beating yourself up about it.

The moment you realized you could celebrate progress instead of punishing imperfection.

The time you said "no" to something because your body, and your boundaries, deserved better.

The moment you realized you're stronger than you've ever given yourself credit for.

You won't find perfection in these pages.

What you *will* find is honesty, humor, hope, and a reminder that your diagnosis doesn't define you.

This isn't a how-to guide written from a mountaintop of discipline.

It's a companion for the messy middle and a reminder that mindset work *is* diabetes work. That real healing isn't just physical, it's emotional, mental, and deeply personal.

I wrote this because I needed it.

And I think maybe you do too.

So let's unlearn the shame, rewrite the story, and walk this road together.

No judgment.

No sugar-coating.

No fake positivity.

Just real talk about getting well, body and mind, while living with type 2 diabetes.

You in?

-Mary

part one
diagnosis, stigma, and speaking up

"Just because someone carries it well doesn't mean it isn't heavy."

— Unknown

You didn't sign up for this, but you *can* own it.

Let's be honest: no one throws a party when they get diagnosed with type 2 diabetes. There's no welcome basket. No empowering orientation. No heartfelt "you've got this!" message tied to your prescription bottle.

What you *do* get is a stack of confusing instructions, a few generic pamphlets, a vague directive to "make lifestyle changes," and the heavy, unspoken suggestion that you did something wrong. You leave the office with questions no one answered, emotions no one acknowledged, and a diagnosis that somehow feels like both a puzzle and a punishment.

This section is here to cut through the shame and the noise.

Because you are not your diagnosis. You're not a failure, a cautionary tale, or a before picture waiting to be fixed. You're a whole person navigating something complicated, and you deserve support, clarity, and a plan that actually works in real life, not just on paper.

Before we talk about blood sugar or food choices, we have to talk about the weight you've been carrying. The shame that crept in before you even understood what insulin resistance was.The outdated myths that still get passed around like gospel in doctor's offices and group chats.

The moment you realized your doctor might not explain what's going on unless you ask.

The way it feels to sit in silence when someone implies that you "should've taken better care of yourself." The guilt that shows up when you're doing your best, but the numbers don't reflect it. And yes, the neighborhood cookout conversations where someone you barely know has the audacity to audit your plate.

We're going to name it all.

Because the silence around type 2 diabetes? It's not helping anyone. And the shame? That's not yours to carry.

This section is about reclaiming your story. It's about understanding your diagnosis on *your* terms, speaking up when something doesn't sit right, and pushing back on stigma, whether it comes from society, your doctor, or that little voice in your head.

You don't need to be perfect. You don't need to prove anything.

But you *do* deserve to be in the driver's seat of your own health.

So let's start there-by separating your self-worth from your A1C, questioning what you've been taught to believe, and reminding you that your story isn't over.

It's just getting a new chapter. And this time, *you* get to help write it.

you are not your diagnosis

. . .

"Your present circumstances don't determine where you can go; they merely determine where you start."

— Nido Qubein

WHEN A DOCTOR TELLS YOU, "You have type 2 diabetes," your whole world doesn't stop, but something inside you might. It's like your brain hits a pause button. Suddenly, you're holding a diagnosis you didn't choose, full of questions no one prepared you for, and trying to figure out what it says about you.

Let me cut through the noise right now. It doesn't say anything about your worth.

You're still you.

The same you from five minutes ago, with a whole, complicated life and a body that has been doing the best it can with the tools, access, and support it had.

But I know how easy it is to slip into shame. I've been there, staring at numbers I didn't understand, and wondering if I somehow "caused" this, replaying every meal, every habit, and every moment like it was going to be used as evidence against me in a trial.

This chapter is here to pull you out of that shame spiral, and to remind you that you are not broken and you are not a flashing warning sign. You are a human being navigating something complex in real time, and you deserve support, clarity, and compassion, rather than blame.

Let's start there.

Been There, Felt That

"I remember staring at my lab results, thinking, 'How did I let this happen?' But the truth is, I didn't let anything happen. I was doing my best with the tools I had. Once I stopped punishing myself, I finally started to heal."

A Personal Note: My Diagnosis Story

I still remember the phone call. It was supposed to be routine blood work for a work physical, nothing urgent or dramatic. So when my doctor said the words "type 2 diabetes," it felt like I got hit by a truck.

I didn't look sick. I didn't feel sick. I was 21 years old and thought I was invincible.

I cried.

All I could think about were my parents, both living with type 2 diabetes, both insulin dependent, both carrying the weight of complications that came from years of struggle. I had front-row seats to their pain. And now I was joining them on stage?

I felt like a failure. How could this happen to me already? I was supposed to be out with friends, not counting carbs and Googling words I couldn't pronounce.

What I wish I had known then, and what I know now, is this:

A diagnosis isn't a punishment. It isn't proof that you've messed up your life beyond repair. It's data, direction, and start of a new chapter, not the end of who you were.

. . .

Reclaiming Your Narrative

So how do you rewrite a story that's been told through blame and shame for decades? Simple. You take back the pen.

You stop measuring your worth by your meals or your glucose readings. And you remind yourself that every body is different, and every journey will be too.

Instead of spiraling into guilt, try asking, "What is my body trying to tell me today?" You start trading criticism for curiosity.

I've watched hundreds of people go from overwhelmed and ashamed to confident and informed. I've seen tears of frustration turn into finish-line smiles. I've seen people come off insulin. I've seen others start insulin and finally breathe easier. Strength looks different for everyone, and all of it counts.

A diagnosis can shake you, but it can also show you possibilities you didn't know were there. Life doesn't end here. It can still be good.

The Identity Trap: You're Not a "Bad Diabetic"

Say it with me: there is no such thing as a "bad diabetic."

You're not a kid getting graded on your lunch choices. You're an adult making decisions in a system that doesn't always give you what you need. Having a rough week, skipping a workout, or forgetting to pre-log your meals isn't failing, and it happens to all of us. But, when we tie our worth to our health, we stop seeing ourselves clearly. What you actually need is grace, support, and a plan that fits your real life, not an Instagram-worthy version of it.

Why Language Matters

The way you talk to yourself shapes how you show up in every part of your life. That voice in your head is the coach you hear most often and if it's filled with blame and shame? No wonder you feel drained before the day even starts.

Practice saying things like:

"I'm learning."

"I'm figuring it out."

"I'm worthy of health, even as I'm growing."

Mindset isn't about putting up a front, it's about choosing words that make space for healing.

———

You're Still the Main Character

If this chapter of your life was a movie, your diagnosis would be the plot twist, not the credits. You're not background noise in your own story. You're the lead. You're the one who keeps showing up, learning, falling, getting back up, and moving forward because you're worth the effort.

Let the world say what it will. Let them catch up to what you already know. You are not your diagnosis. You are your resilience. You are your grit. You are your truth. And no diagnosis can take that from you.

———

What Helped Me Most

What helped me most wasn't a meal plan, a supplement, or a new app. It was learning to separate my worth from my diagnosis.

For a long time, I treated diabetes like a moral report card. High numbers meant "bad." Low numbers meant "good." My A1C dictated my confidence, and every appointment came with a side of shame, no matter what the results were.

The shift began when I learned to pause the judgment. I started asking myself, "Would I say this to someone I love?" The answer was always no.

That's when I began replacing criticism with curiosity. When my blood sugar ran high, I didn't panic. I asked, "What's going on here?" Sometimes the answer was stress, sometimes sleep, and sometimes it was just life. That simple shift gave me power again.

And finding community made the biggest difference. Talking with real people living real lives reminded me I wasn't alone. I wasn't the only one who cried after appointments or skipped checking my numbers out of fear. Those connections helped me remember I wasn't broken. I was learning.

If you're in that place right now, feeling like diabetes has swallowed your identity, please know this: it doesn't have to stay that way. You can reclaim your story one thought, one choice, and one deep breath at a time.

———

grieving the life you thought you'd have

. . .

"You have to let go of who you were to become who you will be."

— Candace Bushnell

NO ONE TALKS about how much grieving comes with a diabetes diagnosis. Not the grief of losing a person, but the grief of losing the version of your life you thought you were going to have.

It's the quiet grief.

The kind that shows up when you're trying to make sense of what this means for your future, your routines, your identity, and your plans, that hits you at random moments because something in your life shifted and you didn't get a vote.

Maybe you expected to feel determined or ready to fight, but instead, you feel cracked open, overwhelmed, confused, or even angry.

And honestly, that makes complete sense.

This chapter exists because grief is part of the human experience. You're adjusting to a new reality, and your emotions are simply catching up. You're not weak for feeling this, and you're definitely not overreacting. You are doing the emotional work no one warned you was part of diabetes care.

Let's name what you've lost and what you haven't.

The Invisible Kind of Grief

Grief has a way of catching you off guard. It shows up in the middle of ordinary moments.

When you realize you no longer trust your body the way you used to, when a friend asks if you want to split dessert and you hesitate, or when you see old photos and remember what it felt like to live without diabetes always humming in the background.

You grieve the simplicity of not knowing and the illusion that you were in control. You grieve the version of yourself who didn't have to explain, justify, or second-guess every choice.

Most of us don't call it grief. We call it frustration or guilt. We tell ourselves to "get over it," to "stay positive," and to "be strong." But grief doesn't disappear just because we refuse to name it. It waits and lingers and begs to be witnessed.

So let's witness it.

Been There, Felt That

"I remember one night, maybe two weeks after my diagnosis, sitting on the couch after everyone else had gone to bed. I had eaten a small, carefully portioned dinner. I tracked everything. I took my medication. I did everything 'right.'

And I still felt awful.

Not physically really, but emotionally. I missed the ease of not thinking so hard and eating without doing math first. And I missed feeling normal, whatever that meant.

So I sat there and cried for the body I didn't trust anymore, the life I didn't ask for, and for the version of me I thought I'd lost.

After that, something changed. I stopped fighting the grief and started honoring it. I let it be part of the process instead of something to hide. Slowly, I began to build something new. Not a perfect version of health, but an honest one, with space for all of it: hope, hurt, strength, softness, progress, and pain."

You Thought It Would Look Different

Maybe you thought this chapter of life would feel easier. That by now you'd be thriving, not adjusting. You'd have more energy, more answers, and more confidence in your health. Maybe you didn't expect to be managing medications, second-guessing dinner choices, or listening to other people's opinions about what's on your plate.

And maybe, deep down, you thought you'd feel more like yourself by now.

That's often the hardest part. It's not just the diagnosis. It's the disruption of identity and realizing that the future you imagined for yourself is going to look different. Not worse. Just different.

Before you can embrace what's next, you have to let yourself mourn what won't be. That doesn't mean giving up or wallowing. It's acknowledging that the life you pictured isn't the one you're living, and giving yourself permission to grieve that without guilt.

Why It Hurts, Even When You're "Okay"

You can be doing everything right: taking your meds, eating balanced meals, checking your blood sugar, exercising and still feel the sadness sitting quietly in the background.

Because grief isn't logical, it's emotional. And living with a chronic condition, especially one as misunderstood as type 2 diabetes, carries a kind of emotional weight that rarely gets acknowledged.

Maybe your diagnosis confirmed your worst fears about your body, or stirred up old wounds about health, control, or self-worth. Or maybe it made you feel like your best days were already behind you.

And maybe the hardest part is that no one else seems to notice you're grieving at all.

But I see you. I know what it's like to hold it together on the outside while quietly falling apart inside, and to smile and nod when someone says "it's manageable," while your brain spins with questions you don't even know how to ask.

If you've been carrying that invisible grief, hear this: it matters. Even if no one else has named it. Even if you've been trying to push through. Even if you thought you weren't allowed to feel it.

You are allowed.

You Don't Need to Rush to Acceptance

Some people will try to hurry you through this. They'll say things like, "It's not that bad," or "At least it's not something worse," or "You just have to stay positive."

They probably mean well, but their words can feel like pressure to skip the messy parts, to perform resilience, and to act brave when what you really need is space and time to feel what you feel.

There's no timeline for this kind of grief. You might feel okay one day and crushed the next. And just when you think you've moved on, you might find yourself overwhelmed again.

That's not weakness. That's being human.

Healing doesn't happen in a straight line and acceptance doesn't magically erase sadness. It just means you're learning to carry it with more grace.

———

What Helped Me Most

What helped me most wasn't pretending to be fine. It was admitting that I wasn't. I had to stop minimizing what I felt and brushing it off as nothing. Because it *was* something. It was loss. Not of a person, but of ease, identity, and control.

Once I let myself feel it, I stopped treating it like a secret.

The turning point came when I called it what it was…grief. Not drama or self-pity. Just grief. I realized I wasn't damaged. I was grieving the life I thought I'd have. And when I gave myself permission to sit with that truth instead of rushing past it, I started to feel a little less stuck.

Talking to others helped, especially those who didn't try to turn it into a silver lining. The ones who simply nodded and said, "Me too." Those conversations reminded me that I wasn't weak for feeling what I felt.

I also stopped trying to "bounce back." Because the goal was never to go back, it was to move forward, slowly, honestly, and with grace. I began building a new kind of normal, where I didn't have to feel okay every day to still be making progress.

Grief isn't something you fix, but something you carry. Over time, it gets lighter, yes, but you also get stronger. And eventually, you find yourself laughing again, hoping again, and living again, not despite the grief, but right alongside it.

———

the stigma problem (and why it's not you)

. . .

"Shame is the most powerful master emotion. It's the fear that we're not good enough."

— Brené Brown

LET'S talk about the elephant in the room: stigma.

It's everywhere.

And if you've ever felt blamed, judged, or misunderstood because of your diagnosis, you're not imagining it.

Stigma rarely shows up as one big event. Instead, it's the collection of small, sharp moments that stick with you. The comments. The assumptions. The side-eye at your plate, or the unsolicited advice from people who don't understand your body or your life. It's the feeling of being judged before you even say a word.

Here's the truth.

The stigma around type 2 diabetes has nothing to do with you and everything to do with outdated, oversimplified stories society keeps repeating.

This chapter is here to help you see that clearly.

Because once you understand where stigma actually comes from, you can stop carrying the shame that never belonged to you.

Let's pull these misconceptions into the light and finally put the blame where it belongs: on the stigma, not on you.

Been There, Felt That

"My coworker looked at my lunch and said, 'Is that okay for a diabetic to eat?' I smiled and said, 'Yes, because I know my body.' But inside, it hit me how exhausting it is to keep defending choices that are nobody else's business."

Where It Comes From and Why It's Wrong

Let's be real about the sources of stigma, because it's not coming from nowhere.

The media has spent decades portraying people with type 2 diabetes as punchlines or cautionary tales. Commercials flash donuts and syringes with dark music, turning a chronic condition into something to fear or mock.

Diet culture tells us that every bite is a moral choice, and if you were just disciplined enough, you wouldn't have diabetes.

Even parts of the medical system can unintentionally add to the shame. Too many of us have been talked at instead of listened to. It's "compliance," instead of collaboration. It's "what did you eat?" instead of "how are you doing?"

And then there's the voice in your own head, echoing everything you've absorbed over the years, whispering, "Maybe I am the problem."

You're not. You're a person navigating a complex condition in a world that barely understands it. That is not the same as being damaged.

. . .

Why Stigma Is Dangerous

This isn't just about hurt feelings. Shame doesn't just stay in your mind. It also seeps into your care.

When stigma takes hold, you might start avoiding appointments because you don't want another lecture, or you might stop tracking food or skip blood sugar checks because you don't want to see the "bad" number. You might stop asking questions or keep quiet about symptoms because you don't want to sound like you've failed.

It's not that you don't care about your health. It's that you've been made to feel like you don't deserve care unless you're getting perfect results.

The fact is, you deserve support no matter what your numbers look like. You don't have to earn compassion by being "a good patient." You get it simply because you're a person.

Unlearning the Noise

You know what starts to break stigma faster than any diet or step count? Talking about it, naming it, and saying, "Actually, that's not true."

Silence breeds shame, and shame keeps us small. But truth sets you free to stand taller.

So let's tell the truth, often and unapologetically.

Type 2 diabetes is influenced by many factors, not just food choices or weight, and managing it is complicated and demanding.

People living with this condition deserve respect, not ridicule.

You don't have to clap back at every comment or give a TED Talk at Thanksgiving. You can simply draw a boundary or change the subject. You can choose when and where to educate others, depending on your energy and peace of mind.

Most importantly, you can stop carrying the shame that was never yours to begin with.

Let's Rewrite the Narrative

The people who make you feel small don't know your story. They don't know what it's like to track numbers, juggle medication, plan meals, fight burnout, and still show up for your life.

But I do. We do.

That's why this book exists…to tell the real story, not the polished pamphlet version. The more we speak up, the more power we take back.

You don't owe anyone proof of your worth and you don't owe anyone an apology for having diabetes.

You are allowed to ask for what you need without guilt, to manage your condition in the way that works for you, and to celebrate your progress, even the parts that don't show up in lab results.

You are not your A1C, a punchline, or a stereotype. You are resilient, real, and rewriting this story one page at a time.

———

What Helped Me Most

What helped me most was realizing that the stigma wasn't mine to carry.

For years, I believed the stereotype. I absorbed every side-eye, every sugar-shaming comment, and every "If you just ate better" remark as if it were gospel. I let it shape how I saw myself. I thought, "If everyone assumes I caused this, maybe I did."

Then one day, it hit me. I was venting to my best friend about how I kept skipping appointments, and I finally said out loud, "I'm embarrassed to go back. I don't want them to see my numbers and think I'm a failure."

That moment shifted my perspective and I realized how wild it was that I felt I had to earn the right to healthcare.

That was the start of the unraveling.

I began paying attention to the voices I had internalized. Whose approval was I chasing? People who had never lived this experience, or my own truth? I learned that shame thrives in silence, and every time I spoke up, even if my voice shook, I reclaimed a piece of myself.

I also stopped feeling obligated to defend my diagnosis. Not everyone deserves an explanation. Sometimes, protecting my peace means simply saying, "I'm doing what works for me," and leaving it there.

What helped most of all was finding people who saw *me*, not my diagnosis, my numbers, or a label, and people who didn't flinch when I shared the messy truth, who reminded me I'm not weak, I'm not to blame, and I'm definitely not alone.

You don't have to carry the weight of stigma any longer. You can set it down and walk forward, free and unashamed.

———

but i don't look sick

. . .

"In the depth of winter, I finally learned that within me there lay an invincible summer."

— Albert Camus

IF I HAD a dollar for every time someone said, "But you don't look sick," I could probably fund my own diabetes research team. It's meant as a compliment, but it lands like a dismissal, as if your experience can't be real unless it comes with visible symptoms.

Living with type 2 diabetes often means living in a body that looks fine to other people while you're managing symptoms, emotions, and decisions they never see. And sometimes, that invisibility feels heavier than the condition itself.

People don't see the blood sugar swings, the exhaustion and the decision fatigue, or the constant adjustments you're making just to feel okay.

This chapter is for every moment you've questioned yourself because someone else couldn't see your struggle.

Your experience is real. And so are your symptoms.

You don't need visible proof to deserve understanding or support.

Let's talk about what invisibility really feels like and why it doesn't make your condition any less real.

The Disconnect Between What People See and What You Live

When you do not look sick, people make assumptions. They assume you are exaggerating or that it's not serious, and that if you just lost weight, followed a diet, or exercised more, everything would fix itself.

They assume it is simple, it's your fault, and that they have the right to weigh in.

And all of that can mess with your head.

When no one sees what you are carrying, you start to question yourself. You wonder if you are overreacting and if you should just be tougher, quieter, or more grateful. You begin to apologize for your boundaries and you start to downplay your needs and shrink simply because you're exhausted.

You begin to doubt your own experience.

Let me remind you of something. Just because it is invisible does not mean it is not real. Just because they do not see it does not mean you are not living it. And just because isn't obvious doesn't mean it isn't valid.

The Medical Side of Invisibility

The invisibility does not stop with friends or family. It can follow you into the doctor's office too.

It shows up when your concerns are dismissed because your numbers are "not that bad, " or when a provider says, "You don't look like a typical diabetic." It shows up when you feel pressure to speak or present yourself in a certain way just to be taken seriously.

Instead of compassion, you get disbelief and instead of support, you get suspicion.

If you do not fit the stereotype, or if you do, it can feel like you cannot win either way. Too healthy-looking to be sick or too big to be trusted. Too calm to be struggling or too well-spoken to be overwhelmed.

So you over-explain or stay silent, hoping one of those approaches will make you heard.

That is a heavy load to carry while you are already managing everything else that comes with diabetes.

Managing the "You Don't Look Sick" Moments

We have all had them, those moments that make you want to scream.

When someone says, "One bite will not hurt."

When a coworker asks, "Are you allowed to eat that?"

When a family member suggests cinnamon pills as a cure.

When a stranger offers advice because they saw a documentary once.

Each comment adds another layer of frustration. You are not just trying to make a healthy choice. You're also trying to protect your boundaries, progress, and confidence. Then someone who doesn't live your reality decides to narrate it for you.

You do not owe anyone an explanation for how you care for your body, and you don't have to educate every person who doesn't get it. You never need to justify your choices to people who aren't living your life.

If it helps, here are a few calm responses to keep in mind:

"Managing diabetes looks different for everyone."

"Thanks for your concern. I have a plan that works for me."

"This approach supports my health right now."

"I don't need advice, but I appreciate your interest."

Sometimes you teach and sometimes you set a boundary and other times you simply walk away. Each option is valid, and each one is strong.

Been There, Felt That

"I will never forget the first time someone said, 'You do not look like you have diabetes.' I think they meant it as a compliment, but it felt like a slap. What did they expect me to look like? What stereotype were they waiting to see?

I laughed it off, but inside I felt defensive. It was as if I needed to prove I was sick enough to justify how I ate, the boundaries I set, or the way I structured my days.

There were so many moments when I stayed quiet just to avoid explaining myself again, but silence didn't help. It only made me feel smaller.

So I started practicing something new: self-trust.

I began validating my own experience instead of waiting for someone else to understand it and I stopped seeking approval and instead focused on what kept me well. Sometimes that meant saying no and sometimes that meant educating people. Sometimes it meant walking away.

I learned that self-trust was more valuable than other people's understanding."

You Do Not Need to Look Sick to Be Taken Seriously

One of the most damaging beliefs out there is that only visible illness is real illness. That unless you are visibly struggling, you must be fine.

But chronic illness does not always announce itself. It shows up in how you eat, sleep, move, think, and plan. It shows up in your lab work, your mental load, and your daily decisions. But it also shows up in fatigue, anxiety, and the constant calculations no one else notices.

You live with that every single day, and it counts.

You do not need to prove your struggle or perform your illness. And you do not need to look sick to deserve care, support, or self-compassion.

What you do need is trust in yourself and in your lived experience. Even if the world cannot see it, you still have permission to rest, protect your peace, and show up for your health in the way you need to.

————

What Helped Me Most

What helped me most was realizing that visibility does not equal validity.

I did not need to be falling apart to deserve care and I did not need to look sick to be struggling. I also did not need to explain myself to anyone to own my truth.

I stopped taking those comments to heart when I finally understood they had nothing to do with me. People speak from their own fear, confusion, or flat-out lack of knowledge. Seeing that made it easier to let go instead of letting it sink in.

I also stopped apologizing for managing my blood sugar in public, for saying no to certain foods, or for honoring my limits. Taking care of myself stopped being something to hide.

And I practiced self-validation. I told myself, "You are doing your best. You know your body. You don't owe anyone proof." The more I said it, the more I believed it.

So if you have ever been made to feel like your condition is not serious enough because you do not look the part, remember this: you do not have to look sick to be worthy of care, compassion, or rest and you do not have to meet anyone's expectations but your own. And you never have to carry your invisible struggle alone.

————

misconceptions that deserve to die out

. . .

"The most dangerous stories are the ones we don't know we're telling ourselves."

— Unknown

LET'S bring some myths into the sunlight.

Type 2 diabetes comes with more opinions and outdated beliefs than almost any other condition, and a lot of them need to go for good.

You've probably heard things like:

"That's the bad kind of diabetes."

"You did this to yourself."

"If you just lost weight, you'd be fine."

"Only older people get that."

None of it is true.

And all of it is harmful.

Misconceptions don't just annoy you. They shape how people treat you, how your doctor talks to you, how you talk to yourself, and how much unnecessary shame you carry for something that was never your fault.

This chapter is here to set the record straight with clarity, honesty, and zero shame.

Let's leave these myths behind so you can move forward with the truth.

Myth One: Type 2 Diabetes Is Caused by Eating Too Much Sugar

This is the classic, original myth that refuses to die.

If sugar alone caused diabetes, every kid who ever ate a bag of Skittles for lunch would be diagnosed before middle school.

Type 2 diabetes is not caused by a sweet tooth. It is a condition rooted in insulin resistance, influenced by genetics, hormones, stress, medications, age, sleep, inflammation, environment, and muscle mass. Yes, food plays a role, but it is not the starring role people assume.

And let's talk about food access. In some neighborhoods, a bottle of soda costs less than a bottle of water. Fast food becomes survival, rather than indulgence. Time, money, and stress all intersect in ways most people never have to think about.

This is not about cupcakes. It's about context.

Myth Two: If You Just Lost Weight, Your Diabetes Would Go Away

Oh, right. Because chasing thinness has always been the secret to healing internal organs.

Weight and insulin sensitivity can be related, but weight is not the whole picture. There are thin people with type 2 diabetes and higher-weight people without it. You cannot look at someone's body and know what is happening inside it.

And while weight loss can sometimes help with management, it is not a cure, and it is not the gold star of health. Most people do not maintain significant weight loss long-term, not because they are lazy, but because biology defends survival.

Let's stop pretending that shrinking your body is the same as healing it. That myth is not only wrong, it's dangerous.

. . .

Myth Three: You Should Be Able to Manage Diabetes with Diet and Exercise Alone

Wouldn't that be nice?

Yes, some people can manage their diabetes through lifestyle changes. And that is worth celebrating. But for most of us, diabetes is progressive. Over time, even when you are doing everything right, your body may still need more help. That might mean medications, insulin, or other tools.

That doesn't mean you failed. It just means your pancreas is getting tired and could use a little help.

Needing support is not a weakness, it's awareness.

Myth Four: Insulin Is a Last Resort

Insulin is not a punishment or proof that you have "let yourself go." It is a medical tool, and one of the most effective ones ever discovered. Since 1921, it has saved millions of lives.

So why do so many people see insulin as a sign of failure? Because the story around it has been warped.

Doctors sometimes hesitate to prescribe it, using it as a threat: "If you don't do better, you'll end up on insulin." Patients delay starting it out of fear or shame. People hide it, worried others will judge them. But insulin itself is not the problem, the stigma is.

Insulin works. It helps you feel better and helps your body function. It is not a last resort, it's a resource.

Myth Five: If You Have Diabetes, You Must Have Done Something Wrong

Let's be crystal clear about this one. Your diagnosis is not a reflection of your character.

Living in a human body in this world, with this food system, this healthcare system, and this level of stress, is complicated. Developing type 2 diabetes does not make you lazy, weak, or irresponsible.

And while we are at it, let's toss out the "good diabetic" versus "bad diabetic" labels. There is no such thing. You are not a walking success story or a cautionary tale. You are a person managing a complex condition the best way you know how.

Been There, Felt That

"After I was diagnosed, I kept wondering if people could see it. I thought maybe they would look at me and think, 'Something must be wrong with her.' It took time, and a lot of unlearning, to realize my diagnosis was not a scarlet letter. It was just one part of a much bigger, stronger story that was unfolding."

What to Do When People Get It Wrong

That part is up to you. Sometimes you educate and sometimes you walk away. Sometimes you channel your inner sassy self and say, "Thanks for your concern, but I'm good."

You do not owe anyone an explanation, but you do owe yourself the truth.

Here's what's true: you did not cause this. You're not failing. You are allowed to ask for help, to use every tool available, and to feel proud of yourself, not despite your diagnosis, but because of how you show up for your health every day.

Let the world keep its myths. You have the facts, the strength, and a whole new story to tell.

————

What Helped Me Most

What helped me most was learning to stop fighting lies with silence.

When I was first diagnosed, I had no idea how much energy I would spend defending myself to strangers, but also to people I loved. I still remember the first time someone asked, "So what did you eat to get diabetes?" Shame hit me like a wave. I smiled awkwardly and changed the subject.

That silence cost me something.

Over time, I realized that misconceptions do not fade because we ignore them. They grow and spread. And worst of all, they start to sink in. I began believing some of those falsehoods myself. When people said, "If you just lost weight, it would go away," or "You shouldn't need meds if you really cared," I absorbed it. I started feeling like I had to earn my health, like I was not allowed to be proud unless I was managing things "the right way."

Eventually, I started reading and talking to people who understood. I got informed, and then I got angry in a productive way. I thought, why am I ashamed of using the tools that help me stay alive? Why am I letting people with no medical background write the script for my life?

That is when I began to respond. Not with lectures, but with clarity. I said things like, "That's a myth," or, "Diabetes is complex, not just about sugar," or simply, "I trust my care plan and my body."

Sometimes I educated and sometimes I walked away. But the thing I did consistently? I stopped shrinking.

What helped me most was owning my truth louder than their ignorance. It gave me freedom and strength. And it reminded me that I did not cause my diagnosis, but I do get to decide how I respond to the noise around it.

You do not have to carry other people's misunderstandings as your burden. Set them down and stand taller. You have truth on your side.

———

advocacy starts with you

. . .

"Speak the truth, even if your voice shakes."

— Maggie Kuhn

YOU LEARN VERY QUICKLY that no one hands you an instruction manual for this diagnosis. Some doctors give you a plan or a pamphlet. Some give you five minutes and a prescription. But very few walk you through how to advocate for yourself, and even fewer teach you that advocacy is a skill you grow into, not something you're supposed to magically know.

Advocacy starts with noticing when something feels off or when you ask a question instead of pretending you understand.

It strengthens the moment you stop apologizing for needing clarity about your own body.

You are allowed to speak up and you are allowed to ask for explanations and you are allowed to say "That doesn't feel right" even if everyone in the room has a degree.

This chapter will help you trust your voice, use it without guilt, and remember that you are the expert on your own lived experience.

Been There, Felt That

"At my very first appointment after getting diagnosed, the nurse handed me a pamphlet and said, 'Just cut back on carbs and you'll be fine.' That was it. No explanation or support. Just a look of pity and a handful of vague instructions. I went home and cried because I felt so lost and overwhelmed. It took me months to realize I had the right to ask for better care. And once I did, everything felt easier to handle."

What Advocacy Really Looks Like

Not everyone feels comfortable speaking up in medical spaces. I know plenty of people who freeze the moment the doctor starts talking. You sit there in that thin paper gown, already vulnerable, while someone rattles off lab numbers or uses words that may as well be another language.

It can feel intimidating. But asking questions isn't rude, it's responsible. Just like requesting clarity isn't overreacting, and saying "I'd like a second opinion," isn't dramatic. Advocacy is about protecting your health.

You are the CEO of your own body. Your healthcare team might be experts in medicine, but you are the expert in you.

Advocacy can sound like:

"Can you explain that in plain language?"

"I'd like to look at other options before adjusting my medication."

"What are the side effects of this, and will it be covered by insurance?"

"I'm not comfortable with that plan. Can we talk through it together?"

These are not demands. They're boundaries, and boundaries are one of the most powerful forms of self-respect there is.

. . .

Advocacy at Home

Advocacy doesn't stop when you leave the doctor's office. It shows up at home, too.

It's telling your spouse, "I need your support, not your food policing." It's explaining to your kids why you check your blood sugar, without making it scary, and it's letting your friends know you'd rather talk about real health than the latest diet trend.

And sometimes, it means drawing a hard line when someone refuses to understand.

You are allowed to say:

"Please don't comment on my plate."

"That joke isn't funny to me."

"I'm doing what works for my body."

You don't owe anyone a TED Talk in return.

Self-Advocacy Takes Practice

The first few times you speak up, it might feel uncomfortable. Your voice might shake, and you might stumble or second-guess yourself. That's okay. Courage lives in the doing, not in perfect delivery.

The more you do it, the easier it gets. You start trusting yourself more and you start expecting better treatment. You begin showing up as someone who knows they matter. Because you do.

I remember one woman from my community who was afraid to ask her doctor about switching medications, even though the side effects were making her miserable. We practiced the conversation during a coaching session. When she finally asked for what she needed, her doctor listened. They adjusted her plan, and she cried happy tears because she realized she could do hard things and still be heard.

That's what advocacy does. It puts you in the driver's seat of your own health.

Advocacy Is a Form of Self-Care

We often talk about self-care like it's face masks and bubble baths, but self-care also looks like refusing to shrink in medical spaces. It looks like pushing back against shame and saying, "I deserve better," and believing it.

Advocacy is self-care because it reinforces your dignity. And in a world that tries to shame people with type 2 diabetes at every turn, dignity is revolutionary.

You don't have to be a policy expert, or need a fancy title or a platform. You just need to be willing to say, "This is my body. This is my health. And I have a say in how it's treated."

That's where you begin taking your power back.

———

What Helped Me Most

What helped me most was realizing I wasn't being difficult, I was actually being brave.

I used to dread doctor's appointments. And it wasn't that I didn't care, I just felt like I wasn't allowed to ask questions. I would nod along, pretending to understand the medical jargon while my mind spun with confusion. When something didn't feel right, I stayed quiet. I didn't want to be labeled "noncompliant," so I left appointments full of doubt and blamed myself for not speaking up.

Everything changed the day I brought a notebook. I wrote down my questions ahead of time because I knew I would freeze otherwise. My hands shook when I pulled it out, but I asked. I interrupted, politely, thank you very much, when something didn't make sense. I pushed back when a plan didn't align with my life.

And guess what? The doctor didn't roll her eyes. She listened and I think she respected me a bit more because I showed up as an active partner, not as a passive patient.

From that day on, I stopped treating advocacy as optional. I treated it as essential.

Advocacy isn't loud or confrontational by default. Sometimes it's as simple as saying, "Can you explain that again?" or "I'd like to try a different approach." And sometimes it's reminding yourself that your health is worth more than being polite.

The same applies at home. Setting boundaries with people you love can be hard, but it's worth it. When I told my family, "No more food jokes at dinner," or "Please stop commenting on what's on my plate," it created space for actual support to grow.

Advocacy helped me breathe again. It gave me back my voice, and once I started using it, everything felt lighter.

You are not being annoying. You are being accountable to yourself. And that matters more than anyone's approval ever will.

———

rethinking your treatment plan

. . .

"If nothing changes, nothing changes."

— Unknown

AT SOME POINT in your journey, you realize your treatment plan is not a fixed thing. It evolves as your body evolves, as life changes, as stress shifts, as hormones fluctuate, and as your support system expands or contracts. The plan that worked last year might not work today, and that doesn't mean you failed. It simply means you're a person with a body and life that's constantly changing.

But here's the tricky part.

We're taught to treat our first plan like the only plan.

We try to force our life to fit a system that stopped fitting us months ago.

This chapter exists to give you permission to rethink the whole thing.

Because your body deserves care that matches who you are now, not who you were when you first got diagnosed.

Let's talk about how to pivot with confidence instead of shame.

Been There, Felt That

"For months, my fasting blood sugars were high even though I was moving more, eating better, and doing everything right. I kept thinking it was me, that I was failing somehow. Then I finally asked my doctor if we could reassess my medication. Turns out, my body just needed more support. It was physiology, not a moral failure."

What a Treatment Plan Really Means

A treatment plan is your full toolkit for managing type 2 diabetes. It includes your medications, how you monitor your blood sugar, what you eat, how you move, how you handle stress, how you rest, and how often you check in with your care team.

It is not a list of rules you have to follow forever. It is a guide that should shift as your body and your life do.

What worked when you were first diagnosed might not work a few months or years later. Hormones, stress, sleep, age, and muscle mass can all influence your blood sugar. If something feels off or your numbers stop making sense, it is not a sign of failure. It is a signal that it is time to adjust.

When to Revisit Your Plan

You know your body best. If your blood sugars are consistently high or low, if your A1C has stopped improving, if you are dealing with unpleasant side effects, or if you have gone through a major life change like surgery, menopause, or increased stress, that is a good time to review your plan.

Feeling unheard, confused, or discouraged is also a sign that something needs to change.

Asking for adjustments is not being difficult. It's being involved.

Your healthcare provider works for you, and your voice belongs in the conversation.

Speaking Up Without Shame

If you have ever thought, *I don't want to seem dramatic,* or *I should just try harder,* you are not alone. But this is not about being dramatic or disciplined. It's about being honest and engaged in your care.

You can say things like:

"I have been tracking my numbers, and they are still high in the morning. Can we look at why that might be?"

"This medication makes me feel sick every day. Are there other options?"

"I have been following my plan, but I am not seeing improvement. What else can we try?"

These are not signs of failure, but examples of good communication. When you bring this kind of feedback to your doctor, you make it easier for them to help you.

Even the most caring doctors cannot know what you are experiencing unless you tell them. They see so many patients every day, and their view of your progress depends on what you share.

Bring your questions, your numbers, and your concerns. You deserve to be heard.

If your doctor will not listen, find one who will. Staying stuck in a plan that is not working helps no one, especially not you.

Medications Are Not a Moral Issue

Starting or changing medication is not a sign that you did something wrong.

You are not weak if metformin is no longer enough, and you're not lazy if your body needs insulin or a GLP-1 medication. You are not a flashing warning sign because your body needs support.

You are doing what is necessary to feel better, stay healthy, and keep showing up for your life, and that's something to be proud of. Medication is a medical decision, not a moral one.

. . .

Define What Health Means to You

Maybe your doctor is satisfied with your A1C, but you still feel tired, foggy, or unsteady. Maybe your labs look fine, but your energy or mood do not. And those things matter too.

Health is not only about numbers. It is also about how you feel in your body, how confident you are in managing your condition, and how much freedom you have in daily life.

You deserve a treatment plan that supports your body and your peace of mind.

A good treatment plan should feel like a partnership, not punishment. If it feels rigid or outdated, or if it leaves you feeling worse, that is your cue to make a change.

You are not being too needy when you ask for better care. You are being proactive and honoring your health.

That is not just healthcare. It's also self-care.

———

What Helped Me Most

What helped me most was realizing that needing more support was not a setback. It was strategy.

For a long time, I thought changing my treatment plan meant I had failed. I assumed that if I needed more medication, it was my fault. If I asked for a new approach, it meant I was not trying hard enough. So I stayed quiet. I stayed stuck on plans that did not work. I stayed on medications that made me feel awful because I did not want to be labeled "that patient."

Things shifted when I finally said, "I don't think this is working anymore."

I had tracked my numbers for weeks and saw the patterns. When I brought my notes and screenshots from my CGM to the appointment and asked about adjusting my plan, my doctor said, "I'm so glad you brought this up." I almost cried with relief.

From that moment, I stopped seeing treatment changes as proof that I had failed. I started seeing them as problem-solving tools. My care plan became a collaboration instead of a command.

I also had to face the emotional side of it. I had to unlearn the belief that more medication meant I was doing something wrong. Once I let that go, the guilt lifted, my numbers improved, and I felt more confident in how I managed my health.

If something feels off, listen to that instinct. Ask questions. Request change. Speak up for yourself even if your voice shakes.

Asking for a new plan is not failure. It is growth, leadership, and it's what thriving actually looks like.

———

explaining type 2 to the world

. . .

"You don't owe anyone an explanation for how you choose to take care of yourself."

— Unknown

THE MINUTE you mention that you have type 2 diabetes, it feels like you've accidentally summoned a panel of experts who didn't get the memo that you weren't taking questions. Suddenly, you're surrounded by the Food Police, the Internet Doctors, and your great-aunt Mildred, who once read an article in Women's World magazine and now considers herself a medical authority.

You didn't ask for commentary on your lunch, or to be a teachable moment. And you certainly didn't ask to become the unofficial spokesperson for a condition that's still widely misunderstood.

And yet, here you are.

Whether it's a coworker side-eyeing your sandwich, a relative asking if you "brought this on yourself," or a friend forwarding the latest cinnamon-sprinkled miracle cure, explaining diabetes can feel like a full-time job you never applied for.

Let's talk about how to explain this condition in a way that protects your peace, honors your truth, and shuts down the noise without draining your energy.

Been There, Felt That

"At a neighborhood potluck, a woman whispered, 'Are you even allowed to eat that?' I just nodded and kept eating. But every comment like that leaves a mark. It's not so much that it hurts my feelings, but it reminds me how misunderstood type 2 diabetes still is, and brings up this feeling of always needing to defend myself and my choices. "

Why You Feel the Pressure to Explain

Part of it is visibility. Diabetes doesn't "look" like anything. People mix up type 1 and type 2, and misinformation spreads faster than truth. And many of us were taught to stay polite, to keep the peace, and to shrink ourselves instead of speaking up.

The other part is that you care. You want to be understood, you want people to have the right information, and you want to manage your health without feeling judged for it.

But here's the thing: You do not owe everyone an explanation. You can choose when, how, and if you share your story. Setting boundaries is protection, not rudeness.

Not every situation needs a deep dive into medical science, but when you decide it's worth explaining, you can do it on your terms.

Keep it simple. You might say, "Type 2 diabetes means my body doesn't use insulin properly. It's more complex than people think, and I manage it with medication, nutrition, and movement." Clear. Kind. Done.

Sometimes, humor works. A lighthearted, "Yes, I can eat that, and no, I won't burst into flames," can make a point without an argument.

And if someone pushes for more than you want to share, redirect without apology. "Thanks for your concern, but I've got it covered." Or, "My care plan is between me and my doctor. Let's talk about something else."

You don't need to justify your choices to anyone who isn't part of your care team or your support system.

When You Don't Want to Explain

Silence is also a valid boundary. You are not a walking public service announcement and you don't owe strangers or coworkers an educational seminar on your condition.

If someone crosses the line, you can say, "I'm not open to talking about that right now," or, "That's personal." Or you can simply change the subject.

Setting limits isn't unkind. It's how you keep your well-being intact.

Family: Where Love and Judgment Collide

Strangers are easy to ignore. Family, not so much. They love you, but their version of "help" sometimes comes out as comments that sting.

You might hear things like, "Should you be eating that?" or, "If you just lost some weight," or, "My coworker's brother did a juice cleanse that cured his diabetes."

When that happens, you have full permission to respond with calm clarity. Try, "I know you care, but this is my body and my decision." Or, "I'm working with my doctor on a plan that fits my needs." Or, "Support means respecting my choices, even when they aren't what you would do."

Repeat these lines until they feel natural. Use them at dinner, in texts, or silently to remind yourself that your boundaries are valid.

Explaining Is Also About You

Sometimes, explaining diabetes is not about educating others. It's about reaffirming your own power and reclaiming your story and reminding yourself that you are informed, capable, and allowed to take up space.

You can say things like, "This is part of my life, but it doesn't define me." Or, "I'm doing what works for me, even if you don't understand it." Or simply, "I'm not here for your approval. I'm here for my health."

These moments are not about winning an argument. They're about standing in your truth.

Here's one you can keep in your back pocket:

"Type 2 diabetes is complex and personal. What works for me might not work for someone else, but I have a plan and a support system. If you're curious, I'm happy to share more, but only if you're open to learning."

Simple. Calm. Firm. And most importantly, on your terms.

You don't have to get every fact right. You don't have to stay composed when someone crosses a line. And you don't have to teach everyone who once Googled "diabetes" how your body works.

You just have to be honest and protect your peace.

Whether that means sharing your story or walking away, that choice belongs to you. You are the expert on your own life and your voice should reflect that.

What Helped Me Most

What helped me most was realizing that I didn't have to educate everyone who had something to say, because not everyone deserves access to my time or energy.

When I was first diagnosed, I tried to be polite. I explained, clarified, and corrected every awkward comment or half-baked suggestion. I gave college-level lectures at Thanksgiving and glucose lectures in the grocery store. And every time I walked away, I felt more drained.

Then one day, I asked myself, *Who made me the diabetes ambassador to the world?*

The answer was no one. I had volunteered for that role without realizing it, and I could quit anytime I wanted.

So I started setting boundaries. I practiced short, calm responses like, "Thanks for your concern, but I've got this," or, "I'm working with my care team on a plan that fits my life." When I didn't feel like explaining, I smiled, nodded, and changed the subject.

And something amazing happened. The more I stopped defending myself, the lighter I felt. The less I over-explained, the more confident I became.

Eventually, I found balance. When someone truly wanted to understand, I shared from a place of strength instead of frustration. I educated without apologizing and I explained without performing.

What helped me most was learning that silence can be just as powerful as speaking up.

I also had real conversations with my inner circle. I told them, "I need your support, not your opinions," and, "Here's what actually helps me." Once those boundaries were in place, I became less defensive and more calm. I no longer felt like I had to prove anything to anyone but myself.

Living with type 2 diabetes is already a full-time job. Explaining it to strangers is optional. You get to protect your peace, and you get to decide who is worth your story.

———

remission vs. reversal vs. reality

. . .

"Success is not final, failure is not fatal: It is the courage to continue that counts."

— Winston Churchill

LET'S clear something up right away: you are not failing if your diabetes isn't "reversed."

There's a lot of noise out there about reversing type 2 diabetes. The idea sounds hopeful and inspiring, but it can also be confusing, guilt-inducing, and misleading.

You've probably seen the headlines:

"Beat Diabetes Naturally!"

"Lose Weight and Cure Type 2!"

"You Don't Need Meds, Just Try THIS One Trick!"

This chapter breaks down the language, expectations, and the reality so you can understand your options without pressure or judgment.

The goal isn't chasing a label. It's building a life that feels steady, sustainable, and supportive.

Let's get clear on what these terms really mean for you.

What "Reversal" Really Means

The word "reversal" gets tossed around far too easily. In medical terms, most professionals are actually referring to remission, which means your blood sugar levels stay in a non-diabetic range without medication for an extended period of time.

That's what people often mean when they say reversal.

It isn't a cure. Type 2 diabetes does not disappear just because your A1C looks great for a while. The underlying issues, such as insulin resistance, remain in the background and can return if management habits stop working.

You did not undo diabetes. What you did was learn how to manage it well, and that is something to celebrate.

Remission can happen. Some people reach it through early intervention, lifestyle changes, or a combination of medication, movement, and nutrition. Sometimes weight loss or surgery helps too.

But remission is not the only version of success.

You can live a full, healthy, joyful life even if your A1C is higher than you want. You can thrive while taking medication and you can make progress without ever reaching remission.

That does not make you less dedicated. It makes you a person managing a complex condition in a complex world.

Been There, Felt That

"When I heard someone say they reversed their diabetes with keto and CrossFit, I panicked. I thought, 'Why didn't I do that? Am I just lazy?' Then I reminded myself that this isn't a competition. My path is mine, and it includes medication, movement, rest, and compassion. That counts too."

Let's Talk About Reality

Here is what is real:

• You can do everything right and still see high blood sugar.

• Stress, hormones, and lack of sleep can raise glucose levels.

• Sometimes medication adjustments are necessary, even after weeks of solid effort.

That doesn't mean you're messing up. It means you're figuring it out like everyone else.

We do not shame people for using blood pressure medication, or tell someone with asthma to "breathe harder." So why do we shame people with diabetes for needing tools that help their bodies work better?

You are already worthy of care, celebration, and respect. No perfect A1C required.

If remission motivates you, that is great, but let it inspire you, not weigh you down with guilt.

Success is not one-size-fits-all. It might look like better sleep, steadier energy, or fewer crashes. It might mean more consistency, better balance, or learning to trust yourself again. Or it might mean asking for help when you need it.

Every bit of progress matters.

Let's stop chasing the fantasy that diabetes can vanish completely because life doesn't work that way.

Reality is learning your body, building habits that last, and giving yourself grace along the way, and creating a version of health that fits your life.

This is not about being perfect enough to reach remission, but about being kind enough to yourself to keep showing up when things get difficult.

You do not need a label to validate your success and you do not need a cure to start living. You're already doing it, one decision, one check-in, and one act of care at a time.

———

What Helped Me Most

What helped me most was letting go of the finish-line fantasy.

For a long time, I thought there would be a perfect moment when everything clicked. My A1C would be flawless, my medications gone, and my numbers steady. I thought remission would be the ultimate proof that I had "won" at diabetes.

Chasing that idea only made me feel like I was always coming up short.

One day, I realized my worth was not tied to whether or not I needed medication. It was tied to how willing I was to keep showing up for myself, even when it was hard.

The shift was seeing diabetes as something I live with, not something I have to beat.

I stopped judging myself for needing support and began asking better questions. Was I sleeping better? Did I have more energy? Was I showing up for my health even on tough days?

If the answer was yes, that was success.

I also learned to tune out the noise. When someone posted about reversing their diabetes, I reminded myself that their story was not my story, and that mine was just as valid.

My success looked like consistency, instead of extremes. It looked like using medication without guilt and celebrating progress that did not depend on perfection.

What helped me most was releasing the pressure to "get rid of" diabetes and focusing on how to live well with it.

Real health is not about reaching remission. It's about reclaiming your power, one honest and consistent step at a time.

———

wrapping up part 1: diagnosis, stigma, and speaking up

"You either walk inside your story and own it, or you stand outside of it and hustle for your worthiness."

— Brené Brown

If you've made it through this first part of the book, pause and take that in. You just did something hard. I don't mean because reading is hard, but facing this stuff is. Looking stigma in the face, telling shame to sit down, and challenging everything you thought you knew about diabetes takes real courage.

When I was first diagnosed, I thought the hardest part would be the food, the numbers, and the meds. And don't get me wrong, those parts can absolutely be overwhelming. But what no one told me was that the real battle would be internal. The judgment, the guilt, and the quiet fear that maybe I did something to deserve this.

This section was about cutting through that noise.

Together, we've called out the BS stories we tell ourselves, corrected the outdated myths people love to repeat, and reclaimed what it means to live with type 2 diabetes on your terms, not the world's.

More importantly, we've started to draw a line between you and your diagnosis. Because you're not just a body to be managed. You're a whole human being worthy of respect, care, and support.

———

What Helped Me Most

What helped me most in those early days wasn't a fancy app or a perfect food log. It was finally giving myself permission to stop feeling ashamed, and to stop treating my diagnosis like a dirty little secret or a life sentence.

What helped me most was learning to ask better questions. And not just at the doctor's office, but of myself. What do I need right now? What am I afraid to say out loud? Where do I need more support?

What helped me most was connecting with other people who *get it*, instead of the kind who try to fix you. Finding the people who will sit with you, cry with you, and say, "Yeah, I've been there too." That kind of connection? That's medicine.

I didn't get better by blaming myself into action. I got better when I stopped believing I had to do it all perfectly to be worthy of care. You're allowed to be a work in progress and still demand support.

And if nobody's told you this today: You're doing better than you think.

———

And now, we move forward.

Part 2 is all about the mindset shifts that make this life not just manageable, but meaningful. It's about emotional resilience, motivation that lasts longer than a motivational quote, and learning to treat yourself like someone worth showing up for (because spoiler alert: You are).

So take a breath. Drink some water. Shake off whatever stories you're still carrying about who you should be.

Because we're not doing "should" anymore. We're doing truth, growth, and maybe a little stubborn joy.

Let's keep going.

part two
mindset shifts
and mental health

"You can't heal the body without healing the mind."

— Dr. Gabor Maté

Blood sugar isn't the only thing that needs balance.

You can count carbs, take your meds, walk after every meal, and still feel like you're stuck in a mental tug-of-war with diabetes. Why? Because living with type 2 isn't just a physical challenge, it's an emotional one, too.

No one tells you how personal this gets. That it's not just about numbers on a meter, but it's about the story you tell yourself when those numbers aren't where you want them to be, the pressure to be "good" all the time, the guilt when you're not, and the way your brain can spiral from one high reading into a full-blown downward spiral.

It's about the voice in your head that whispers, *"You should be doing more."*

The one that turns every setback into a character flaw, that tells you you're either on track or off the rails, and never in between.

This section is where we untangle all of that.

It's where we get honest about perfectionism, people-pleasing, burnout, and fear. And where we stop pretending motivation is some magical unicorn that shows up when you need it.

It's where we talk about what it really takes to change your mindset, without toxic positivity, without using good vibes to gaslight yourself, or pretending a vision board can fix your pancreas.

Because the truth is, mindset isn't a side dish. It's the whole dang plate. It's the foundation of your transformation.

It's what everything else, food, movement, medication, and self-care-*sits on.*

We're not here to sugarcoat it (pun absolutely intended).

We're here to shift the way you see yourself, your progress, and your potential.

I'm not saying mindset fixes everything, but without it, none of the rest stands a chance.

So if you've ever felt like you're doing everything right and still losing steam, hey friend, you're in the right place.

If you've ever sabotaged your own success, abandoned your goals, or wondered why consistency feels so hard, you're not damaged. You're "normal". And you're not alone.

Let's talk about the stuff that actually keeps you going when motivation doesn't and what it really means to care for your whole self.

Ready? Let's do this.

the fear of success (yes, it's real)

. . .

"What if I actually get what I want...and I still don't feel good enough?"

— Unknown

LET'S get one thing straight: being afraid of failing makes sense. That's been drilled into us since the third-grade spelling bee, the missed free throw, and the "better luck next time."

But being afraid of succeeding? That's the plot twist no one talks about. And yet, it's real. Sneaky. And ridiculously common.

We talk a lot about self-sabotage like it's laziness or lack of willpower, but sometimes it's actually a fear response. Success shakes the ground you've been standing on. It forces you to rewrite your story. And when that story has always been one of struggle, the idea of "better" can feel almost threatening.

You don't recognize yourself in ease. You don't know what to do with peace, so you brace, you downplay, and you hide. You might tell yourself, *Don't get too comfortable,* even when that comfort is what you've been fighting for.

. . .

When Success Feels Like a Threat

Here's how it shows up in real life.

You finally find a rhythm that feels good. Maybe your blood sugar steadies, or your clothes fit differently, or you wake up with energy and maybe, just maybe, a little pride. And then out of nowhere, panic sneaks in.

But it's not because it isn't working…it's because it *is*.

That little voice starts chattering:

What if I can't keep this up?

What if people expect more from me now?

What if I change too much and lose part of who I am?

What if I get better and I still don't feel happy?

You start picking yourself apart, and looking for cracks in the progress. You question if it's luck, if it's sustainable, or if it's even real. That's your brain doing what it was designed to do, protecting you from the unknown.

Even when the unknown is *feeling good*.

Why It Happens

When your identity has been built around struggle, peace can feel suspicious. Like stepping into bright sunlight after too long in the dark. You squint, you flinch, and you wonder what's waiting to go wrong.

For years, I had wrapped my worth in trying, fighting and constantly starting over. I was the "comeback story," the "resilient one," the woman who *never gave up*. That identity served me when I needed grit, but when things started finally *working*, it backfired. Because if I wasn't struggling, who was I?

It seems a little backwards because it's not that you don't want success. It's that success threatens the story you've always told yourself.

Maybe that story sounds like:

I'm the one who always has to fight harder than everyone else.

Struggle makes me strong.

Ease means I'll let my guard down and lose it all.

That's not weakness, it's conditioning. You've been rewarded for enduring, not for receiving, and for pushing through, not for pausing. For surviving, not thriving.

So when ease shows up, you don't trust it.

Been There, Felt That

"I've lived that cycle of panic.

There were times I'd hit a milestone, whether it was a lower A1C, dropping a pants size, or simply feeling better in my own skin, and instead of celebrating, I'd start pulling back.

I'd tell myself, Don't say anything. Don't post it. Don't jinx it.

I'd smile politely when people complimented me, but in my head, I was already listing the ways I might mess it up.

Part of that fear came from how others responded to my progress. Some people celebrated me, but others got quiet. A few even made comments like, "Must be nice," or, "I could never do that." And suddenly I was the one making myself small so no one else would feel uncomfortable.

Being stuck started to feel safer than being seen. Because visibility brings expectations, and opinions, and pressure.

But here's the truth I had to face:

Playing small doesn't protect you.

It just keeps you invisible."

What If You Let It Be Easy?

So here's your permission slip to let success feel safe.

You're allowed to get better without explaining it to everyone, to have a good day with your numbers and just enjoy it, and to be proud without apologizing for it. You don't have to downplay the good to stay relatable. And you don't have to shrink your joy to make others comfortable.

Success doesn't mean you've signed up to be the valedictorian of type 2 diabetes. Or that you have to maintain perfect numbers or never have an off day again. It just means something is working.

And you deserve to know what *working* feels like.

How to Move Through the Fear

Start by noticing it. When the panic shows up, pause and ask, *What am I really afraid of here?*

Often, the answer isn't failure. It's visibility, responsibility, or loss of control. And once you name it, it loses its grip.

Then, celebrate without disclaimers. If your A1C improved, don't water it down with, "It's still not where I want it." Just say, *I'm proud of this*. Period. You earned that moment.

Talk to your fear out loud. Maybe even write it down.

"I'm afraid I won't be able to keep this up."

Then imagine your best friend said that to you. What would you tell her? Probably something like, *You don't have to be perfect. You just have to keep showing up.*

Redefine success while you're at it.

Success isn't about being perfect forever. It's about making aligned choices more often than not and coming back when you drift.

And remember, rest is part of the plan. You don't need to "earn" your progress with constant hustle. You're allowed to have ease, too.

For many of us, healing is learning how to hold good things without flinching.

It's trusting that peace doesn't mean the other shoe is about to drop, and realizing that ease is not the enemy of growth, but the reward for it.

When I finally stopped waiting for something to go wrong, I started noticing everything that was right. My mornings felt lighter, my meals felt less like math problems and more like nourishment, and my workouts became moments of gratitude instead of punishment.

And the irony? That's when I made the most consistent progress of my life. Because I wasn't chasing success anymore, I was living it.

Success isn't a finish line. It's a feeling.

And you are allowed to feel good, even while you're still growing.

—————

What Helped Me Most

There was a moment, right in the middle of progress, when I looked in the mirror and actually felt proud. My numbers were down. I felt strong. I could walk up a flight of stairs without losing my breath.

And almost instantly, fear barged in.

What if I can't maintain this? What if I backslide? What if people expect more of me now? Who am I if I'm not the one always fighting?

That joy was immediately shadowed by panic. I realized I'd been living in survival mode for so long that peace didn't feel safe, it felt foreign. Somewhere along the line, I'd learned that getting better meant constantly raising the bar until rest was impossible.

So I started to unlearn it.

I stopped trying to "hold on" to success and started to *live* in it.

I shifted my definition of success from something I had to earn and protect to something I could experience and expand. I didn't need to prove I could stay perfect, I just needed to stay curious, honest, and kind to myself when things got shaky.

When fear crept in, I repeated a simple mantra:

"I can enjoy what's working without fearing it will disappear."

Because joy counts. Rest counts. Celebrating your own progress counts.

Healing isn't just about what you do when things go wrong. It's also about what you allow when things go right.

—————

comfort zones, chaos, and why getting stuck makes sense

. . .

"Growth and comfort do not coexist."

— Ginni Rometty

LET'S BE HONEST: sometimes the "comfort zone" isn't comfortable at all. It's just familiar.

It's the place where you know what to expect, even if what you expect isn't great. The place where you sigh and say, "I know this isn't ideal, but at least I know how to handle it."

We are wired to cling to predictability. Our brains love patterns and routines, even when those patterns quietly drain us. Sometimes the comfort zone isn't cozy. It's a decorated cage so we hang up a few motivational quotes, throw a blanket of routine over it, and call it safety.

I've lived there. I've nested there.

For a long time, I told myself I was being realistic, when really, I was just tired and scared. I wasn't preserving peace. I was protecting predictability. And what I was actually doing was settling for stuck.

. . .

Resistance Isn't a Character Flaw. It's a Clue.

If you've ever been told you're "set in your ways," let's call it what it usually means:

"I know this isn't working, but change feels hard, and I'm exhausted."

That doesn't make you lazy or unmotivated. It makes you real.

But resistance isn't the enemy, it's information. It's your brain waving a little flag that says, "Something about this feels unsafe." Even when the change is something you want, doing things differently can feel like stepping off solid ground.

Sometimes that resistance shows up quietly. You swear off exercise because you're "not a gym person," even though you've never tried movement that actually feels good in your body. You resist a medication conversation because you think you should be able to do this on your own. You cling to a food plan that worked twenty years ago, even though your hormones, stress, and lifestyle have changed completely. Or you convince yourself you can't walk at lunch, can't meal prep, can't adjust your schedule, because the chaos you're already in feels familiar.

Sometimes being stuck means talking yourself out of even trying.

I've done that too. There were seasons when I stayed loyal to what wasn't working simply because I knew what to expect. Same routine. Same frustration. Same results. At least it was predictable. Change felt like risk, and risk felt scarier than staying stuck.

Why We Stay Stuck (Even When We Want More)

Resistance doesn't always shout, sometimes it whispers.

"It won't work for me."

"It's too late to start over."

"I don't want to get my hopes up again."

Those thoughts don't come from nowhere. They usually come from real disappointment. Maybe you've been burned before by a plan, a program, or a promise that didn't deliver. Maybe you're grieving the body you used to have, the energy you once felt, or the simplicity of life before everything got so complicated.

Sometimes our identity gets tangled up in the struggle. You've been the one who's "trying," the one who's "working on it," for so long that success feels foreign. Even positive change can feel threatening when it disrupts the inner status quo.

Familiar feels safe, even when it hurts.

The Comfort and Chaos Loop

But comfort doesn't work alone. Chaos loves to jump in.

You know the loop. Life is busy, stressful, unpredictable, so you wait.

After the holidays.

After this deadline.

After things calm down.

Except they never really do.

Chaos will happily keep you company for years if you let it. It tells you, "Now isn't the right time," and because you're tired, you believe it. Comfort keeps you still. Chaos keeps you spinning. Together, they create that exhausting state of almost starting.

You see it when you keep setting goals but never following through. When you tell yourself you'll "start fresh Monday," every Monday. When you avoid checking your numbers because you just can't deal right now. When you know what works, but you avoid it anyway.

That loop feels safe, but it quietly erodes your confidence. Every time you repeat it, it reinforces the belief that maybe change just isn't for you. But that isn't truth. It's habit. The good news? Habits can change.

When Fear Dresses Up as Logic

Fear is sneaky because it rarely introduces itself honestly. It doesn't say, "I'm scared." It says, "This probably won't work anyway," or "I've tried before," or "It's just not the right time."

Fear loves to dress up as truth. It sounds reasonable, analytical, and protective. But logic that keeps you frozen isn't logic. It's protection gone rogue.

You don't have to believe every thought you think. You can pause and ask, "What if it's okay to try anyway?"

That small question is often where courage begins.

Discomfort isn't danger. It's data. It's your body and brain learning something new in real time.

That uneasy feeling when you do something different isn't a sign you're failing. It's a sign you're stretching. Growth doesn't require bulldozing your life or torching your comfort zone to the ground. Sometimes growth is about editing, not erasing.

Ask yourself:

What parts of my routine still serve me? Keep those.

What feels heavy or outdated? That's where change belongs.

You don't need a total overhaul. You need one intentional shift. One walk after dinner. One honest blood sugar check. One medication conversation. One moment of rest without guilt.

Discomfort doesn't mean you're doing it wrong. It means you're learning.

Been There, Felt That

"I remember a week when I decided to stop waiting for motivation and just test a theory instead. There was no grand plan and no miracle routine. I promised myself I'd move for ten minutes a day, however that looked.

Some days it was walking around the kitchen while the coffee brewed. Some days it was stretching before bed. It felt laughably small at first, until it didn't.

After a few days, those ten minutes stopped feeling like an obligation and started feeling like a reset button. I wasn't rebuilding my whole life. I was just creating a small opening for something new.

That's when it clicked. Momentum doesn't start with massive effort. It starts with one small tweak to what's already familiar."

―――――

What Helped Me Most

There was a stretch where I kept saying, "I'm trying," but nothing was actually changing. I was doing what I'd always done: tracking, cutting, pushing through workouts that punished my body instead of supporting it. When it didn't work, I blamed myself instead of questioning the method.

The shift came from one question:

"What if this isn't failure? What if it's feedback?"

I stopped fighting my body and started listening to it. I swapped punishment for partnership. I traded intensity for movement I could actually enjoy. I talked to my doctor instead of white-knuckling side effects. And I scaled down instead of quitting.

I didn't erase everything I'd done before. Instead, I evolved it.

What helped me most was realizing that my way wasn't the only way. And when I let go of that story, things felt lighter. My energy. My body. And my outlook.

Growth didn't start with discipline or motivation, but with permission to let go of the old and try again, only smaller this time.

Because real growth doesn't happen when life gets easy. It happens when you stop confusing familiar with safe and choose one honest step forward anyway.

———

the emotional
weight of weight loss

. . .

"You are allowed to love yourself and want to feel better at the same time."

— Unknown

LET'S talk about the *other* kind of weight.

Not the one your doctor charts in a file, and not the one that makes your jeans tight.

I'm talking about the emotional weight…the identity shift and the mental load of trying to shrink your body in a world that already tries to shrink your worth.

When you live with type 2 diabetes, the topic of weight loss gets complicated fast. You're told it's the answer to everything: your numbers, your energy, your confidence, and your health. But the truth is, it's never *just* about the number on the scale. It's tied up in years of messages about what's "good," what's "healthy," and what's "enough."

And when the weight does start to change, that comes with its own set of emotions. Pride, pressure, fear, and confusion, sometimes all at once. Nobody tells you how heavy that part can be.

You're told that losing weight will fix everything. It'll fix your blood sugar, your self-esteem, and your life.

But what if it doesn't?

What if you lose the weight and still don't feel at home in your body?

What if you get healthier but find yourself terrified of gaining it back?

What if people treat you differently and you don't know how to handle it?

This is the part that doesn't make it into the pamphlets. It's the part that shows up in the quiet moments, in dressing rooms, at family dinners, and in the space between pride and panic.

The Truth Behind the Compliments

You start hearing it: *"You look amazing!" "What's your secret?" "I didn't even recognize you!"*

And maybe part of you glows with pride. You've worked hard, and it feels good to finally be seen.

But then another part whispers, *Why does my worth seem higher now that my weight is lower?*

It's a strange mix. Validation and unease all tangled up together. Because now what? Do you have to maintain this new version of yourself to stay "amazing"? What happens if you gain a few pounds? Do the compliments disappear? Does your value disappear with them?

That's when body image and identity collide. You start to wonder if people like you *more* now, and what that says about how they saw you before. But even harder, you start to wonder what *you* believed about yourself before.

I remember how jarring it felt when people's attention suddenly shifted. The same people who once overlooked me were suddenly full of praise and curiosity. It was validating, but it was also disorienting. Because while my body was changing, my insecurities hadn't caught up yet.

Been There, Felt That

"I lost the weight. Everyone noticed. Everyone praised me. But when the noise quieted, I was still stuck in fear: scared to eat, scared to regain, and scared I still wasn't enough. That's when I stopped chasing approval and started fighting for something bigger...my peace, my trust, and a life I didn't have to shrink to make myself and others comfortable."

What Diet Culture Forgot to Mention

Diet culture sells weight loss as the destination, like the pot of gold at the end of the rainbow.

But here's the uncomfortable truth: weight loss isn't always healing.

Sometimes, it's just trauma in a smaller pair of pants.

Because if you never felt safe in your body to begin with, shrinking it won't magically change that. If you grew up in a home where food was love or punishment, or where your body was policed, weight loss can stir up all kinds of old pain.

Even when the intention is health, the process can awaken grief for the person you used to be, the comfort foods that once connected you to your family, and the version of yourself who didn't overthink every bite.

That doesn't make you weak or ungrateful. It means you're finally doing the *emotional* work that wellness actually requires.

I've seen so many people chase smaller bodies thinking peace lives there, but peace doesn't live in a pant size. It lives in the way you speak to yourself.

Your Body Isn't a Project

Let's get one thing straight. You're allowed to pursue health and still reject the idea that your body is a problem to solve.

Health is a practice, not a punishment. Your body isn't a report card or a test of willpower. It's the home you live in and it deserves care, not constant criticism.

You don't have to "deserve" your body. You don't have to earn rest, joy, or confidence through struggle. And you certainly don't have to apologize for taking up space. Not now, or ever.

You're allowed to want to feel stronger without obsessing over being smaller, to enjoy food without turning every meal into math, and to feel good in your body without chasing the version that lives in a filtered photo.

The scale has been sold to us as a truth-teller. But it's not truth. It's data. Incomplete data at that.

If you're taking your medication consistently, moving your body more, sleeping better, feeling more confident, managing stress, or simply showing yourself kindness, that's progress, even if the number doesn't change.

The scale might catch up or it might not. But you are still healing. You are still improving your health, your mindset, and your relationship with yourself.

You are still winning.

For a long time, every weigh-in felt like judgment day. I'd wake up, hold my breath, step on the scale, and let that number determine whether I was "good" or "bad" that day.

It didn't matter that my blood sugar was stable, that I was sleeping better, or that I had shown up for myself all week. One number could erase all of that in seconds.

That kind of emotional whiplash doesn't just affect your mood, it changes the way you live. You start avoiding social events, skipping meals, and overcorrecting after one "bad" day. The emotional weight becomes heavier than the physical one.

But the truth is, no number can define your effort, your worth, or your progress.

———

What Helped Me Most

What helped me most was realizing I had handed over all my power to a machine. A piece of plastic and metal was deciding how I felt about myself.

So I took my power back.

I didn't smash the scale or declare war on it. I just stopped letting it speak louder than I did. I started asking myself better questions.

Did I have more energy today?

Did I move my body with gratitude instead of punishment?

Did I treat myself with respect?

Did I feel grounded and calm instead of reactive and restricted?

Those became my new measures of progress.

And I started noticing new kinds of wins:

I walked past a mirror and didn't flinch.

I ordered lunch without pulling up an app.

I wore the damn bathing suit.

I gave myself grace for an off day and got right back to living.

And here's the beautiful part...My health still improved. My A1C went down, and my confidence went up. But most importantly, I stopped waiting to feel good about myself until the number agreed with me.

Because here's what no one tells you...weight loss might change your body, but healing your relationship with your body changes your life.

When I started focusing on sustainable habits, emotional balance, and self-respect instead of constant restriction, everything got lighter. Not just my body, but my heart.

I didn't need to earn my own care. I just needed to give it.

You don't have to wait until your body looks a certain way to treat it like it matters. You can love it into health instead of punishing it into submission.

That's what helped me most.

———

from burnout
to boundaries

. . .

"Almost everything will work again if you unplug it for a few minutes, including you."

— Anne Lamott

LET'S TALK BURNOUT.

Not the "I stayed up too late scrolling" kind.

The deep, soul-heavy, everything-feels-like-too-much kind.

The kind that sneaks up on you after months or years of doing your best. After tracking, planning, adjusting, advocating, and holding it together. The kind that shows up when you're tired of deciding what to eat, tired of checking numbers that don't seem to cooperate, tired of thinking about diabetes at all, and tired of pretending that it doesn't take up mental space.

Diabetes burnout doesn't happen because you're weak or lazy or indifferent.

It happens because you're living in a body that never gets a day off.

There is no finish line here. No graduation ceremony. No point where someone taps you on the shoulder and says, "You're good now, you can stop paying attention." Even when you're doing everything "right," your body still has a mind of its own. Stress, sleep, hormones, illness, work, family, and life don't politely wait their turn. They pile on.

Burnout is what happens when the effort never lets up, but the relief never comes.

And here's the part no one really prepares you for. Burnout doesn't always look like drowning your struggles in a pint of ice cream. It's not always tears on the kitchen floor or a full-blown breakdown. Sometimes it's quiet. Sometimes it's numb. Sometimes it looks like avoidance, resentment, or that heavy sigh you let out when your monitor beeps again.

It might look like skipping blood sugar checks because you already know the number won't be good. Taking your medication late or not at all because you're just so over it. Avoiding appointments because you don't want another lecture. Turning off alerts because one more reminder feels like too much.

Sometimes it sounds like, "I'll get back on track Monday."

If that feels familiar, you are not alone. You're also not a failure or lazy or unmotivated. You are burned out.

Burnout is not a character flaw. It's the natural result of carrying a chronic condition in a culture that praises pushing through and rarely talks about what it costs.

Most burnout follows a familiar pattern. You leave an appointment fired up, scared, or both. You decide this time you're going to do all the things. Track everything. Move more. Eat better. Hydrate. Sleep. Stay positive. Be consistent. Be 'good'.

And for a while, it works.

Then life shows up. A kid gets sick. Work explodes. Your numbers go sideways for reasons no one can explain. You miss one check-in, then another. Suddenly you feel behind. Shame creeps in quietly and whispers, "See? You can't keep this up."

Before you realize what's happening, you're not just tired. You're numb.

But that numbness isn't failure. It's a signal. It's your system saying, "Something has to change."

Been There, Felt That

"I kept thinking if I just pushed harder, things would get better. But all that got better was my ability to pretend I was fine. My blood sugar was up, my mood was down, and I snapped at my kids because I hadn't done anything for myself in weeks. My 'aha' moment was realizing I didn't need more discipline. I actually needed more boundaries."

Burnout isn't just about diabetes tasks. It's about everything layered on top of them. The expectations. The emotional labor. The pressure to be the "good" patient. The constant explaining. The advice you didn't ask for. The guilt that shows up when you choose rest instead of productivity.

You can't manage a chronic condition while managing everyone else's expectations first. That's not resilience. That's martyrdom. And burnout will always collect its payment.

This is where boundaries come in.

Most of us don't burn out because we don't care enough. We burn out because we care deeply and protect ourselves poorly. We say yes when we're exhausted. We over-explain. We keep showing up for everyone else while quietly disappearing from ourselves.

Boundaries aren't walls. They're fences that keep your peace intact so you don't lose yourself tending to everyone else's wants and needs.

A boundary doesn't require a long explanation or a permission slip. It might sound like, "I don't discuss my medication choices." Or, "I'm not taking health advice from people who don't live in my body." Or, "I'm logging off early tonight because what I need isn't another podcast episode about productivity. It's rest."

If setting limits makes you uncomfortable or guilty, it probably means you were taught that your needs should come last. But you don't owe anyone your burnout to prove your commitment to your health.

Rest deserves its own rebrand here too. We live in a culture that treats exhaustion like a badge of honor. Burnout has been dressed up as hustle, and collapse disguised as dedication. But rest isn't quitting. Rest is recovery.

If your health journey feels like a second full-time job, it's okay to renegotiate the terms. Ask yourself what's actually sustainable. Going all-in for two weeks and crashing, or going steady for months without losing yourself in the process?

How to Come Back to Yourself

Coming back from burnout doesn't mean doing more. It means doing less with intention.

That starts with naming it. Saying, "I'm burned out," isn't admitting defeat. It's telling the truth, and truth creates space for change.

You don't have to fix everything at once. You don't have to disappear from your care to take a break. You can step back without stepping away. You can shrink the task until it feels manageable. Drink water when you wake up. Check your blood sugar once today. Eat something steady, not perfect. Rest when your body asks. Text someone who gets it and say, "I'm struggling."

Those small acts aren't failures. They're lifelines.

Pay attention to your early warning signs. Irritability. Brain fog. Snapping at the dog. Crying over expired lettuce. When those moments show up, pause. Ask yourself what your body is asking for. Then listen before you hit empty.

Burnout thrives in silence. It convinces you that everyone else has it together and you're the only one falling apart. That's a lie. Community matters. Being seen matters. Support matters.

You are allowed to pause. You are allowed to rest. You are allowed to protect your peace.

Just don't disappear from yourself.

———

What Helped Me Most

What helped me most was realizing burnout wasn't a moral failure. It was feedback.

For a long time, I believed success meant being relentless. Tracking everything. Logging every bite. Smiling through it all. One morning, I stared at my meter and thought, I can't do this today. I just felt empty. Completely exhausted by the thought of it.

I was afraid to admit it. I thought saying "I'm burned out" would make me look weak. Instead, it opened the door to empathy, understanding, and real help.

I stopped chasing perfect days and started aiming for okay ones. I focused on what actually brought me peace. Water. Quiet mornings. Sitting outside on my porch. Checking my sugar once instead of five times.

I began saying no without explaining myself. I scheduled rest the same way I used to schedule workouts. I made a list of minimum-effort wins for my hardest days. Drink water. Take meds. Walk for five minutes. Breathe.

The biggest shift was this: I stopped believing I had to earn rest by burning out first.

Seeing rest as a requirement instead of a reward changed me. Sustainable wellness doesn't come from pushing harder. It comes from treating your peace like it's part of your treatment plan.

Because it is.

You don't have to be perfect.

You just have to keep coming back.

———

the perfectionism trap

. . .

"Perfectionism is just fear in a fancy outfit."

— Elizabeth Gilbert

LET'S just get this out of the way:

If you've ever said, *"I'll start over Monday,"* this chapter is for you.

If you've ever had one bite of dessert and thought, *"Welp, the day's ruined, might as well finish the cake,"* this chapter is for you.

And if you've ever felt like "being good" meant being hungry, tired, and cranky, but still forced yourself to hit 10,000 steps while fantasizing about throwing your Fitbit across the room, then this chapter is *definitely* for you.

Welcome to the perfectionism trap.

It's sneaky because it starts out looking like motivation. It sounds responsible, disciplined, even noble. You set out to "do better," to "get healthy," and to "finally follow through." But somewhere along the line, your good intentions get hijacked by shame, comparison, and a twisted form of control that looks like discipline but feels like desperation.

Suddenly, you're not trying to *feel well*, you're trying to *perform wellness*. And perfection will always make you feel like you're losing.

Been There, Felt That

"I once skipped dinner at a friend's house because I was scared I'd eat something 'off plan.' I sat in my car afterward and cried. I didn't cry because I'd 'saved' myself from calories, but because I was lonely, hungry, and tired of being at war with food. That's when I realized perfection wasn't protecting me. It was isolating me."

The "Good Girl" (or Guy) Effect

Perfectionism often starts with praise.

You get applauded for how "disciplined" you are, how "good" you've been with food, or how much weight you've lost. People cheer for your control, your willpower, and your results. It feels good, because who doesn't like gold stars?

But then life gets lifey. You skip a workout. Your blood sugar spikes. Or you eat pasta because you're exhausted and need comfort. Suddenly, the applause stops. You don't get celebrated for rest, recovery, or moderation. You get silence.

And that's when perfectionism tightens its grip. It says, *You only get praised when you're good. You only matter when you're "on."*

So you chase that next perfect day like a hit of validation, and you keep chasing it until you forget how to feel good without earning it first.

Perfectionism teaches us that worth is conditional, that only our highlight reels count, and that anything less than flawless means failure.

But that's the lie.

The Food Confessional

If you grew up in a world that moralized food, good vs. bad, clean vs. dirty, you probably know this one well.

You eat pizza and feel like you've sinned. You skip dessert and feel righteous. You log your meals like confessions: *Forgive me, Coach, for I have eaten carbs.*

That mindset is exhausting. It keeps you locked in a cycle of guilt and repentance that has nothing to do with health. Food isn't a test of your morality. It's fuel, culture, and connection.

When I finally started untangling morality from meals, I realized something. I'd been using perfectionism as a shield. As long as I was being "good," I didn't have to face the real work of learning to trust myself.

The All-or-Nothing Trap

Perfectionism doesn't believe in middle ground.

You're either fully on track or completely off. You're either "good" or "bad." You're either winning or worthless.

That's why so many of us get caught in the endless cycle of "starting over." Because perfectionism doesn't leave space for being human.

But here's the truth: there is no wagon to fall off of. There's just *you*: showing up, learning, adjusting, and trying again.

Real change happens in the gray areas. Change is showing up in the days that aren't perfect, but still count and in the moments you give yourself grace and keep going anyway. That's where sustainability lives and that's where healing actually sticks.

You don't need more willpower. You need more compassion.

Perfectionism says, *Try harder.*

Compassion says, *Be kinder.*

You can't punish yourself into wellness. You can't hate yourself into health. You can't chase perfection and peace at the same time.

So when things go sideways, pause instead of pouncing. Ask, *What do I need right now?* And not *What did I mess up?*

Let your goals be flexible, not fragile.

Measure your progress by how supported you feel, instead of how perfect you performed.

Because the truth is, most of us don't need another rule, we need relief.

The Burnout Behind "Being Good"

There's a quiet kind of burnout that comes from living in "on plan" mode. It's the exhaustion of constantly managing every bite, every step, and every choice like it's a test. It's waking up each day already behind.

I lived there for years. I told myself I was being "disciplined," but I was really just terrified of losing progress, being judged, and of failing publicly.

It took time (and a lot of humility) to realize that chasing perfect wasn't making me healthier. It was making me miserable.

———

What Helped Me Most

I spent years trying to "get it right." The right food. The right plan. The right body. I was convinced that if I could just be *good enough* for long enough, I'd finally arrive at that magical finish line where everything clicked.

But perfectionism doesn't have a finish line, it just keeps moving the goalpost.

Every time I "slipped," I felt like I had to start over. One imperfect meal, one missed workout, one high blood sugar, and I'd spiral. The shame hangover was heavier than any actual setback.

What helped me most was realizing that the goal isn't perfection, it's resilience.

So I started measuring progress differently. Instead of measuring it by how many days I stayed "on plan," I measured it by how quickly I could recover when I wasn't. It stopped being about how few treats I allowed myself, but by how easily I could enjoy one without guilt. I stopped judging myself by how flawless my week looked, but by how kind I was to myself when it didn't.

I replaced *perfect* with *consistent, starting over* with *staying in it,* and *shame* with *strategy.*

And when I stopped tying my worth to how "good" I was at being healthy, I found something I'd been chasing for years…peace.

Now, I treat myself like someone I trust, and someone I'm rooting for, who deserves care even on the messy days. And that shift didn't just make wellness possible, it made it personal.

———

comparison is a confidence killer

. . .

"Don't compare your chapter one to someone else's chapter twenty."

— Unknown

IT SNEAKS IN UNEXPECTEDLY.

You're feeling pretty good about your day. You got your movement in, you made a mindful food choice, and you even remembered to check your blood sugar without spiraling into judgment. Things are humming along…until you pick up your phone.

And there it is. A post from someone in your group who just dropped three clothing sizes, or an old friend running a half-marathon, or someone sharing their A1C like it's a gold medal.

And just like that, everything you were proud of feels small.

Comparison doesn't walk in and announce itself. It slides in sideways. It whispers, *She's doing better than you. You should be further along by now. You're behind.*

It turns your wins into not-quite-enoughs.

It turns celebration into shame, and sometimes it turns community into competition.

And if you let it take root, it can completely derail your progress because comparison told you, whatever progress you were making? It didn't count.

Why Comparison Hits So Hard in Diabetes

Managing type 2 diabetes comes with a lot of data: numbers, charts, percentages, and goals. And in a world obsessed with tracking and progress and "hacking" everything, it's easy to fall into the trap of thinking you're only as successful as your most recent reading.

Add to that a culture where social media is filled with curated snapshots of people's best moments, and suddenly, you're surrounded by highlight reels that look like reality.

You see someone's "perfect" plate and think, *I didn't eat that clean today.*

You see someone's workout stats and think, *I didn't push that hard.*

You see someone say they're off medication and think, *I must be doing something wrong.*

But here's what you're not seeing:

The days they didn't share.

The mornings they cried.

The weeks they plateaued.

The guilt they carried.

The support they had, or didn't have.

Comparison is a confidence killer because it strips away all the nuance and context and convinces you that your struggle is a sign of failure instead of *proof* that you're showing up for yourself.

Different Bodies. Different Diagnoses. Different Lanes.

You wouldn't compare how fast a car moves through traffic to how a bike handles a mountain trail. Different vehicles. Different terrain. Different mission.

And yet, we constantly compare bodies, lifestyles, responses to treatment, and timelines. As if we're all working with the same genetics, resources, hormones, history, mental health, support systems, medications, access to care, and lived experience.

Spoiler alert: we're not.

You might have weight loss resistance, insulin resistance, a hormonal imbalance, depression, an injury, trauma responses, cultural expectations, caregiver responsibilities, or all of the above.

Of course your journey looks different. It *should*.

But instead of acknowledging that truth, comparison convinces us that there's a "right" pace. A "right" number. A "right" outcome. And if you're not hitting it fast enough or loud enough, you must not be trying hard enough.

Let me be clear: That is a lie.

There is no universal timeline for healing.

There is no gold star for doing it faster.

And there is no shame in moving at the speed of *what's sustainable*.

You're not late, and you're not behind. You're right on time for your life.

The Inner Comparison Nobody Sees

There's another kind of comparison we don't talk about enough and that's the kind you do inside your own head.

The version where you compare who you are *right now* to who you used to be.

You think about the "old you". Maybe before your diagnosis, before the weight gain, or before life got heavy. And instead of holding her with compassion, you use her as a weapon.

I used to be more motivated.

I used to run 5Ks.

I used to be able to wear that.

I used to care more.

But that version of you existed in a different season. She had different challenges, and she wasn't carrying what you're carrying now.

And chances are? She wasn't as "together" as you remember her to be.

Sometimes we glorify the past because it gives us something to measure against. But if looking back only ever makes you feel small, it's not reflection, it's sabotage.

You don't need to become the old you.

You need to become the version of you who no longer uses shame as a motivator, who honors what her body can do now, and who leads with trust not comparison.

What If You Measured Progress Differently?

What if the metric for success wasn't a number or a weight or a pant size, but peace?

What if you celebrated showing up for your walk *even when you didn't feel like it?*

What if you gave yourself credit for logging your numbers, even if they weren't what you hoped for?

What if you paused to notice that you don't spiral into guilt like you used to?

That counts.

That's progress, and that's healing.

We've been trained to look for visible, measurable change. But some of the most powerful shifts happen internally, quietly, in the way you talk to yourself and treat yourself when no one's watching.

Been There, Felt That

I used to spiral constantly when I saw other women posting progress. Sometimes it was weight loss. Sometimes it was blood sugar wins. Sometimes it was just how confident and consistent they seemed. And no matter how much I had accomplished, I'd start questioning it all.

Was I doing enough?

Was I behind?

Why didn't it look that easy for me?

I'd scroll through groups and feel smaller and smaller, until I wasn't proud of anything I had done. Just ashamed of everything I hadn't.

Even my own memories became comparison traps. I'd think about the version of me who hit a certain goal or crossed a finish line and instead of cheering her on, I'd turn her into evidence that I'd somehow gone backward.

But over time, I learned to recognize comparison for what it was: a distraction, a lie, and a detour that pulled me off my own path.

And I started talking back.

I'd look at someone else's post and say, *Good for her. And I'm doing great too.*

I'd catch myself in the mirror and think, *This is what effort looks like.*

I'd remember that every chapter of my story has built the strength I have now.

I stopped chasing a version of success that wasn't meant for me, and I finally felt free.

––––––––

What Helped Me Most

What helped me most was recognizing when I was falling into the trap before I drowned in it. I started noticing the physical signs: tight chest, anxious scrolling, mood shifting after seeing someone else's win. Instead of letting those feelings spiral into shame, I started asking: *What am I making this mean about me?* That question alone was a game-changer.

I also learned to get honest about context. I reminded myself that I don't know what someone else is dealing with. I don't know their medications, their history, their stress levels, or their access to care. And I stopped assuming their win meant something about *my* worth.

Eventually, I built a habit of self-acknowledgment. Before I looked outward, I looked inward. What was one thing I was proud of? What was one way I'd shown up for myself that day? I didn't wait for validation, I gave it to myself. And slowly, that built a kind of confidence comparison couldn't touch.

So if you've been stuck in that loop: comparing, doubting, shrinking, I want you to know…it's not a character flaw. It's just a mindset that needs a reset. And you have full permission to opt out of the race you never intended to run. Your path is yours, and it's worth celebrating.

———

motivation is a liar (and why you don't need it)

. . .

""You don't rise to the level of your motivation. You fall to the level of your systems."

— James Clear

LET'S start with some truth. Motivation is like that old college roommate who still owes you rent and only shows up when there's wine or something fun to do. It's exciting at first and it gives you all the feels when you're watching a transformation video or planning a brand-new routine.

And then it disappears. Usually by day three.

If you've ever said, "I'll start Monday," only to wake up Monday with zero interest in starting anything except another Netflix series, you're not alone.

This chapter is about breaking up with motivation, or at least learning to stop waiting for it to appear. Because it won't. Motivation is unreliable. It comes and goes with your mood, the weather, and how much sleep you got last night.

News flash: it's not coming to save you.

84

Been There, Felt That

"I used to get hyped on Sundays. I'd write an intense meal plan, schedule workouts down to the minute, buy all the veggies, and swear this time was different. By Wednesday I was exhausted, annoyed, and mad that I wasn't suddenly a new person. I'd skip a workout, grab a snack that wasn't 'on plan,' and everything would unravel. It took me forever to realize motivation wasn't the problem, my expectations were."

Motivation Is Mood-Based, and Moods Change

Motivation depends entirely on how you feel, and feelings shift constantly. Everything influences it. Your blood sugar, sleep, stress, hormones, and even someone microwaving fish in the office can affect how much energy you have to care.

If your action plan depends on feeling motivated, you'll stay stuck. Motivation is unpredictable, and building your life around it is a setup. It doesn't care about your goals or what you need to get done.

That's a problem when you live with type 2 diabetes, because your health doesn't wait until you "feel like" checking your blood sugar. It doesn't wait for the right playlist, the right weather, or the perfect day. And you can't wait either.

Discipline Over Motivation

Let's clear something up. Discipline is not punishment. It's not yelling at yourself to do better. It's brushing your teeth, feeding your dog, or plugging in your phone before bed. You don't wait to feel motivated to do those things. You do them because they matter.

That's what real discipline looks like. It's quiet, steady, and dependable.

Checking your blood sugar. Taking your medication. Choosing breakfast that keeps you steady instead of spiking your glucose. None of that requires excitement. It just requires follow-through. Motivation is emotion, while discipline is structure. And structure is what carries you when motivation fades.

Making It Easier to Show Up

Real talk? I have never once felt excited to strength train. Not once. But I still do it because I know what happens when I don't. My body stiffens, my energy drops, and my blood sugar gets harder to manage.

So I stopped waiting for motivation and started designing for ease. I lay out my workout clothes the night before, make playlists that make me laugh, and combine movement with things that lift my mood, like sunlight or a good podcast.

Movement doesn't come from motivation. In fact, it's the opposite: Motivation comes from movement.

Action first. Feelings follow.

When you show up before you feel ready, you prove to yourself that you can take action even when it isn't convenient. And that's real power.

The Myth of the Spark

We love to chase that spark, the sudden burst of energy that makes us want to overhaul everything at once. But sparks fade. And when they do, most people stop. It's not because they're weak, they were just never taught that consistency is quieter than excitement.

No one stays hyped up forever. The people who seem endlessly motivated aren't running on adrenaline. They've simply built habits that keep them steady when that initial excitement fades.

If motivation is the spark, discipline is the pilot light that keeps the fire going.

Building Momentum Without the Mood

Instead of waiting to want to do something, start small. Tell yourself you'll do it for five minutes. Walk for five. Stretch for five. Prep one meal. Most of the time you'll keep going, but even if you don't, you've still done something. Action *always* beats intention.

Pair new habits with old ones. Take your meds when you make your coffee. Check your blood sugar after brushing your teeth. Linking new actions to routines you already have creates rhythm instead of resistance.

And on the rough days, when you're tired or overwhelmed, go back to the basics. One veggie. One short walk. One deep breath before dinner. You don't have to do everything. You just have to stay connected.

When You Don't Feel Like It Is When It Matters Most

Anyone can show up when it's easy, but the real growth happens when you do it anyway.

It's simple to move your body when the music hits and you're feeling good. But on the days when you're exhausted or frustrated, that's when your future self starts whispering, "Thank you for showing up."

Trust is built through those moments, not in the exciting ones. Trust grows in the quiet consistency that no one sees.

———

What Helped Me Most

There was a time when I believed motivation was the missing piece. I told myself, "If I could just get back in the zone" or "If I could just feel like it again." I waited for the spark to come back while scrolling through other people's highlight reels, or saving Pinterest inspirational quotes hoping it would rub off. It never did.

Then one day, I realized motivation wasn't coming. No song, no quote, no perfect timing was going to save me. If I wanted to feel better, I had to move first, even if it felt awkward or boring.

So I started small. One short walk. One meal I didn't overthink. One blood sugar check I didn't judge. No hype. No "starting over Monday." Just quietly showing up consistently.

Little by little, I began trusting myself again. Each small action proved that I could keep going, even on days I didn't feel like it.

What helped me most wasn't inspiration. It was creating systems that worked when I was tired or unmotivated. It was remembering that my health depends on what I do in the messy middle, not on how fired up I feel at the start.

Now, when someone says they're waiting for motivation, I smile and tell them to stop waiting and just start walking. One step is enough. Even if you grumble through it, movement changes things.

Because once you move, something shifts. You build momentum and confidence. And one day you realize your life doesn't rely on hype or vibes or timing. It runs on care, consistency, and self-respect.

You don't need to feel ready. You just need to remember why it matters.

———

visualization, vibes, and victory laps

. . .

"Your brain believes what you consistently tell it. So let's start telling it something that serves you."

— Unknown

LET'S BE HONEST: most of us have rolled our eyes at the words *visualization* or *positive mindset*. Especially when we're juggling work, managing meds, trying to keep blood sugar steady, and wondering if we drank enough water today.

The last thing anyone wants to hear after a hard day is, *"Just picture success and it'll happen!"*

Ma'am, I pictured myself eating a salad yesterday and still ended up demolishing a plate of nachos.

So let's be clear. This chapter isn't about pretending everything is fine or slapping glittery affirmations over your struggles. It's about using real mindset tools that actually work. The tools that help you *retrain your brain* to stay grounded and capable when life (and your blood sugar) gets messy.

Been There, Felt That

"I used to roll my eyes at affirmations. Like really? I'm supposed to tell myself I'm powerful while I'm crying in the car after a rough doctor's appointment? But the first time I pictured myself actually handling a hard moment with compassion instead of spiraling, I felt it. And once I saw it in my mind, I started believing I could do it in real life."

What Visualization Really Does

Visualization isn't magical thinking. Think of it like mental rehearsal. It's not "manifestation" in the sparkly, wish-upon-a-star sense. It's the same brain training athletes, performers, and leaders use to build confidence before big moments.

You imagine yourself doing the thing *before* you actually do it, which helps your brain recognize it as familiar instead of threatening.

It's like a dress rehearsal for your real life. Picture yourself checking your blood sugar calmly instead of dreading the number. Imagine yourself choosing a walk when the couch is calling. See yourself saying, *"No thanks,"* to the food that leaves you sluggish and choosing something that supports you instead.

When you can see it, your brain starts to believe it.

And when your brain believes it, your body follows.

When the Vibe Is Trash

Real talk-some days, the vibe is *not it.*

You're tired, frustrated, and over it. The last thing you want to do is visualize anything except crawling into bed.

But visualization isn't about being in a good mood. Instead, it's about creating a little space between you and the chaos and picturing a calmer response before your emotions take the wheel.

When everything feels off, try asking yourself, *"What would the kindest version of me do next?"*

Then, picture that version of you taking one small action like drinking a glass of water, taking one deep breath, or checking your blood sugar without judgment.

You don't have to feel inspired. You have to imagine yourself steady, and then do one small thing to match the picture in your mind.

Mindset work isn't about turning bad days into good ones. Instead, it's about helping you feel anchored inside the bad days so they don't sweep you away.

The Power of Pre-Paving

Pre-paving is one of my favorite visualization tools. Think of it as leaving sticky notes for your future self. It's you, mentally preparing for what's coming so it doesn't catch you off guard.

Before a family dinner, picture yourself choosing food that helps you feel balanced, without guilt or restriction. Before a doctor's appointment, imagine sitting calmly, notebook in hand, asking questions confidently instead of nodding through confusion. Before the weekend, picture yourself feeling rested and proud because you made choices that actually support the life you want.

When you mentally rehearse moments like that, your brain starts to feel safe in them. And when your brain feels safe, your choices start to feel easier.

This isn't "hocus pocus." It's neuroscience. And it works.

———

What Helped Me Most

I used to think mindset work was fluff, like motivational slogans trying to dress up a blood sugar crisis with butterflies and rainbows. But what changed my perspective was using visualization as *prep*, instead of pressure.

Before difficult conversations with my doctor, I'd picture myself sitting there calmly, asking real questions instead of pretending to understand. Before holidays, I'd imagine myself surrounded by food and laughter, making a choice I could feel good about.

That mental rehearsal helped me respond instead of react. It gave my brain a script to follow when things felt chaotic.

But what helped me most was learning to celebrate my effort instead of perfection. I started tracking what I called my "mindset wins", not numbers, or macros, or calories, but moments of self-trust.

Like choosing water and noticing my energy improve.

Or skipping the guilt after resting instead of pushing through.

Or pausing before emotional eating and giving myself grace whether I followed through or not.

Those moments rewired my thinking. They helped me believe I was someone worth showing up for, even on the days motivation was nowhere to be found.

And once I believed that, the other 'stuff' got easier.

———

the mindset shift that changed everything

. . .

"You can't hate yourself to wellness. You have to love yourself there."

— Me

IF YOU'VE BEEN LIVING with type 2 diabetes, or honestly, just living life in a body that doesn't always cooperate, you probably know the internal soundtrack by heart.

"I should've done better today."

"Why can't I just get it together?"

"If I had more willpower, this wouldn't be so hard."

These thoughts sneak in quietly. They sound reasonable, responsible, even. But here's what no one tells you when you're first diagnosed: that voice in your head, the one that narrates every bite, every test result, and every skipped workout, can shape your health just as much as your blood sugar monitor or your medication can.

You can white-knuckle your way through a new diet for a few weeks and you can track your numbers perfectly, but if the internal dialogue underneath it all is still running on guilt and shame, the crash is inevitable. Eventually you'll stop, and you'll think it's because you're weak, but really, it's because constantly checking, tracking, and correcting wears on even the strongest people. The problem isn't you.

It's the script you've been working with.

The Shame Loop

Shame has mastered the art of disguise. It pretends to be discipline. It masquerades as motivation, and it tells you, *"I'm just trying to keep you accountable,"* when really, it's eroding your confidence.

Shame whispers:

"You're a bad diabetic."

"You ruined everything by eating that."

"Your numbers are high, which means you're failing."

It feeds off silence. The more you isolate, the louder it gets. It convinces you that your mistakes are proof you're defective, not proof you're learning.

And shame is sneaky because it doesn't always announce itself. Instead, it hangs out quietly behind every "I'll start again Monday."

I once heard someone describe shame as "the hand on the back of your neck pushing your head down." That's exactly how it feels when you're living with a chronic condition that's constantly judged by numbers and outcomes. You start to believe your worth lives in those numbers too.

But here's the truth: if shame worked as a strategy, we'd all be world-class athletes with perfect A1Cs and endless willpower. Shame doesn't drive long-term success, it only drives hiding, exhaustion, and rebellion.

The Myth of Tough Love

I used to think being hard on myself was the same as being responsible. If I let myself off the hook, I'd lose control. So I'd double down. Every "mistake" became a lecture and every high blood sugar became a moral failing.

And sure, that mindset kept me in line for about five minutes. Then it would backfire spectacularly. Listen, fear might fuel a few early wins, but it can't sustain a lifetime of self-care.

Tough love works only when love comes first. Otherwise, it's just toughness.

Real accountability doesn't sound like, *"You blew it again."* It's, *"You can do better, and I believe you will. Now let's figure out how."*

Self-Compassion: The Most Misunderstood Skill

People hear "self-compassion" and picture bubble baths and soft music. But compassion isn't just pampering, it's discipline with a bit of heart.

It's the voice that says, *"You matter too much to keep treating yourself like this."*

It's giving yourself a second chance before the shame spiral starts, and it's taking a deep breath, collecting data, and moving forward without the added trip on the downward spiral.

There's solid research behind it: people who practice self-compassion after setbacks are more consistent with medication, more resilient under stress, and less likely to quit. When you feel safe with yourself, you stop wasting energy on self-criticism and start using it to actually change.

Compassion doesn't let you off the hook, but it does end the cycle of punishing yourself for being human.

Rewriting the Script

Most of the harsh lines in your head didn't start with you, they were handed down.

Maybe from a rushed doctor who focused more on numbers than humanity, a family member who equated discipline with deprivation, or from a culture that praises weight loss no matter what the cost.

Those voices blend together until you can't tell whose they are. But most likely, they're not yours, and they're not facts.

You get to write a new script.

Start by catching the old dialogue in action, and noticing it without judgment: *There's that voice again, telling me I'm failing.* Then ask your-self, *Would I say this to someone I love?* If not, it's not fit for me either.

At first, rewriting feels awkward, like learning a new language. But the more you practice, the more fluent you become. Eventually, kind-ness becomes your default. Choosing kindness doesn't mean every-thing is perfect, but that you're finally learning to trust yourself to handle things, even when it's not.

Been There, Felt That

"On a visit to my endocrinologist, the doctor walked in the room and asked how I was. I replied with the standard, "good" and I'll never forget his response. He said, "If you were good, your A1C would be under 7." As if a higher A1C was the deciding factor on whether I was good or not. I never saw that doctor again."

———

What Helped Me Most

There was a time when I believed the only way to stay on track was to stay hard on myself. I mistook cruelty for control and I thought guilt was fuel.

But beating myself up didn't make me disciplined, it made me feel discouraged.

The shift came when I started asking better questions instead of assigning blame. When my blood sugar spiked, I stopped saying, *"What's wrong with me?"* and started asking, *"What happened here?"*

Sometimes the answer was practical: stress, lack of sleep, or a meal that didn't balance right. Sometimes it was emotional: loneliness, frus-tration, or fear. Either way, curiosity gave me something shame never could, information.

And information leads to action.

I began treating my numbers as conversation starters instead of verdicts. A high reading didn't mean failure; it meant my body was asking for support. Drink water. Take a walk. Adjust. Move on. No punishment required.

I also started expanding my definition of success. Some days, success meant eating a balanced breakfast. Other days, it meant checking my glucose even when I was afraid of the result. And sometimes, success meant forgiving myself before the guilt set in.

The real magic happened when I finally internalized that my worth wasn't on trial. It wasn't tied to my numbers, my weight, or my discipline level. My worth was constant, unshakable, even on the messy days.

Everything felt lighter after that. And ironically, that's when my health actually improved. Because consistency follows compassion. You stop swinging between extremes and start living in the middle, where balance, sustainability, and peace live.

Now, when I hear that old inner critic gearing up, I remind it: *We don't talk like that anymore.* I don't need fear to keep me in line. I need faith in the version of me who's still showing up.

And that's the mindset shift that changed everything.

You don't have to bully yourself into progress. You can love yourself there with one gentle thought, one kind decision, and one brave, imperfect day at a time.

———

taking the long way home

. . .

"Healing is not about changing who you are; it's about changing your relationship to who you are."

— Suzanne Heyn

LIVING with type 2 diabetes can sometimes feel like you've been dropped into a lifelong scavenger hunt you never signed up for. Everywhere you turn, someone has an opinion about what you *should* be doing whether it's the next diet, the newest medication, or the miracle fix. There's a constant soundtrack of judgment and expectation telling you that you're not doing enough, or that if you just tried harder, you'd be "better."

It's exhausting, overwhelming, and sometimes, it's paralyzing.

So let's take a collective deep breath and ask a different question:

What if the goal isn't to "win" against diabetes?

What if the goal is simply to *live*? And I mean living well, fully, and on your own terms.

Navigation not Failure

The language we use around diabetes often sounds like a war zone. We "fight" the disease, we "beat" cravings, and we "conquer" blood sugars. But here's the truth: you're not at war with your body. You're in a relationship with it, and like any long-term relationship, it can be complicated.

Some days you're in sync. You eat well, you move your body, and you feel amazing. Other days, your blood sugar's a roller coaster, your energy's gone, and you're just trying to get through dinner without crying into your salad.

Trying to defeat your body is a losing game. You waste energy fighting yourself instead of working with yourself, and that's never the path to healing. The point isn't domination, it's collaboration.

Your body isn't the enemy. It's the partner that keeps showing up, even when you're frustrated with it, even when you've ignored it, and even when it's sending you messages you'd rather not hear. You're both learning each other's language. And that process is navigation, not failure.

Been There, Felt That

"I used to think I had to 'beat' diabetes every day. That if I didn't, I was losing. But I finally realized it's not about winning, it's about living. Now, I see my CGM like a weather app. The numbers shift just like the forecast, but I use that info to keep moving forward instead of freaking out."

This Is a Long-Term Relationship, Not a Crash Diet

Somewhere along the way, we were taught that managing diabetes is about perfect discipline: perfect tracking, perfect meal prepping, and perfect numbers. But perfection is a trap and it's the fastest route to burnout.

True progress doesn't come from rigid control. It comes from *adaptability*. It's learning when to push and when to rest and understanding that success looks different on Tuesday than it did on Monday. It's realizing that long-term consistency will always matter more than short-term intensity.

When you stop expecting perfection, you make space for peace.

There's no finish line in this work and definitely no final exam that proves you've "passed" diabetes. And that's actually freeing. It means you don't have to rush. You don't have to fix everything by Friday. You get to build something sustainable instead of chasing something temporary.

The long way home might not be glamorous, but it's the one that lasts.

You Deserve a Life, Not Just a Plan

When you were diagnosed, you probably got a stack of pamphlets, a lecture about carbs, and maybe a follow-up appointment. What you didn't get was a manual for how to *live* with this. How to manage the emotional weight, the daily decisions, and the invisible exhaustion of thinking about blood sugar every single second of every single day. Rinse. Repeat. Forever.

So let this chapter be your permission slip.

You're allowed to have good days and hard days. You're allowed to feel proud one minute and angry the next, and you're allowed to say, "This sucks," without guilt or explanation. You can rest without calling it quitting and you can pause without labeling it a setback.

You don't have to earn your right to live well by achieving a perfect A1C. And you don't have to be the poster child for diabetes wellness to deserve joy, confidence, or a second helping of watermelon in July.

Your worth isn't on a sliding scale with your blood sugar. Your worth is fixed, permanent, and nonnegotiable.

This journey isn't about winning or losing. It's about building a life where you're no longer fighting yourself. It's about trusting your body, trusting your process, and trusting that you're not behind.

Because there is no behind when the only finish line is *living*.

The hardest part about taking the long way home is that it doesn't always look like progress. Some days, it feels like walking in circles.

You take your meds, you eat the salad, and you do everything "right," and your numbers still spike.

That's the part that breaks people. It's the moments when you're doing all the work and it's still hard. But here's what I've learned... those are the moments where growth is happening underneath the surface.

Progress in this journey is rarely linear. It's messy, winding, and often invisible until one day you look back and realize, *I'm handling things now that used to break me.*

That's the quiet miracle of consistency, and that's the reward of patience.

What Helped Me Most

When I finally stopped treating diabetes like an opponent to defeat, everything softened. My daily routines became less about punishment and more about partnership.

Instead of asking, *"Am I doing enough to beat this?"* I started asking, *"How can I work with my body today?"* Some days that meant getting outside for a walk even when I didn't feel like it, and other days, it meant choosing rest without guilt.

I stopped making decisions out of fear of judgment, fear of failure, or fear of complications, and started making them out of love for my future self, and for the body that's still trying its best, even on the days I'm frustrated with it.

I began celebrating my choices instead of obsessing over outcomes and I started treating high blood sugars as information instead of indictments. I learned that I could hold two truths at once: I am both a masterpiece and a work in progress.

I realized that my blood sugar didn't have to be perfect for my life to be good, and that joy and stability could coexist with imperfection. And I learned health isn't a test to pass, but rather a relationship to nurture.

Every time I chose curiosity over criticism, I felt lighter, and every time I practiced compassion instead of control, I trusted myself a little more.

And that's how it happens: slowly, steadily, one intentional step at a time. You start by managing your condition, but eventually, you build a life where it no longer defines you.

Diabetes becomes just one *part* of your story, not the whole story.

So if you take nothing else from this chapter, take this:

You are not failing. You're finding your way. And the long way home still gets you home.

———

your why (and how to find it again)

. . .

"When you feel like quitting, remember why you started."

— Unknown

AT SOME POINT in this journey, you probably felt that spark and the moment you decided things had to change. Maybe it was a scary doctor's appointment, or a tough conversation with someone you love, or maybe it was just a quiet moment in your kitchen, realizing you were tired of your own excuses.

Whatever lit that first fire, it meant something. It gave you a reason to start showing up for yourself again. But somewhere along the way, after the doctor visits, the meal plans, the medication changes, and the everyday life stuff, that reason can fade into the background.

Life gets loud. Work, family, stress, and fatigue…they all pile up, and suddenly you're not fueled by purpose anymore, you're running on autopilot. You start doing the things because you "should," not because you *want* to. And slowly, that spark starts to dim.

When that happens, you're not lost. You're disconnected from your "why."

But the beautiful part? You can always reconnect.

. . .

Why the "Why" Matters

Your "why" is the heartbeat behind every healthy choice you make. It's the thing that carries you through the days when motivation ghosts you, when progress feels invisible, when your blood sugar won't behave and you're wondering why you bother.

But here's the catch: your why isn't a number.

It's not your A1C or the size of your jeans. It's not how many carbs you tracked or how many steps you logged. Those are results, data points, not desire points.

Your *why* is deeper. It's personal.

It's wanting to walk your grandkids to the park without needing to rest halfway.

It's picturing yourself dancing at your child's wedding, laughing without worrying about crashing later.

It's feeling strong enough to say yes to things again: to life, to adventure, and to joy.

Your why is about being present in your own story, not performing for someone else's version of "good enough."

When the Spark Fades

Losing sight of your why doesn't happen overnight. It fades slowly. You get tired, you juggle too much, you hit a plateau, and you start questioning whether any of it's worth the effort.

You tell yourself you'll "get back to it" when life calms down, but life doesn't calm down, it just continuously changes shape.

Losing your why doesn't mean you've lost your drive. It means you've been in survival mode too long, and survival mode is not where purpose lives. It's where fatigue and frustration grow.

Losing your why doesn't mean it's gone forever. It's still there, waiting underneath the noise, and ready to be rediscovered when you slow down long enough to listen.

Been There, Felt That

"My wake-up call wasn't dramatic. I was eating junk in the kitchen after the kids went to bed (again) and it hit me: I was choosing momentary comfort over being here for the people I love most. That night, I made a decision. My kids were going to see me fight to stay alive. Not just survive, but live. That became my why. And it's the reason I keep showing up, even when it's hard."

Reconnecting with Your Why

When your purpose starts to blur, the first step is to zoom out. You can't see the big picture when you're stuck staring at the smallest details: numbers, data, and to-do lists. Ask yourself, *"If everything felt a little easier tomorrow, what would that look like?"* Maybe it's energy to take a walk after dinner, or not dreading the doctor's office. Maybe it's peace.

Once you can see that image, lean into the feelings it gives you. Your true why should move you, not guilt you. If your why feels like pressure, it's probably a "should" dressed up as purpose.

Then, make it visible. Don't trust your tired brain to remember it on a hard day. You've got to write it down. Put it on your mirror, your phone, your fridge, your journal, or all of the above. Seeing your why reminds you that you're not just working toward numbers, you're working toward *meaning*.

Let Your Why Evolve

The why you started with might not be the one that fits you now, and that's a good thing.

At first, a lot of us begin with fear: *I don't want complications. I don't want to get worse.*

But over time, that fear-based why can burn you out, because it's heavy and unsustainable.

As you grow, your why can shift into something softer and richer: *I want to feel proud of myself again.*

I want to experience life without limits.

I want to love the body I'm in, even while I'm still learning how to care for it.

You're not inconsistent for changing. You're evolving, and every new season of life deserves a new reason to keep going.

Your Why Is an Anchor

When progress feels slow and frustration hits hard, your why is what steadies you, and what keeps you from giving up when the results don't come fast enough or when life throws a curveball.

You don't need endless willpower or perfect discipline. What you need is an anchor. Something that holds you steady when everything else tries to pull you under.

And that anchor doesn't have to be epic, but it does have to mean something real to you.

It might be a photo of your grandkids on your fridge, or a note on your phone that says, *"You promised yourself better."* Or maybe it's a simple phrase you whisper when you want to quit: *Remember why you started.*

Your why is stronger than your excuses, but it needs space to breathe, and it's up to you to give it that space.

————

What Helped Me Most

For a long time, my "why" was fear. Fear of everything related to this disease: fear of complications, fear of failure, fear of not being around for the people I love. But fear doesn't sustain you. It burns hot, fast, and out.

The shift happened when I traded fear for love.

Love for my future self who wants to dance at weddings, travel freely, and watch my family grow.

Love for my body, the one that's kept showing up for me, even when I was too angry or ashamed to show up for it.

Love for the life I'm still building, not the one I thought I lost the day I was diagnosed.

Once I made that shift, staying connected to my journey felt natural. I stopped chasing perfection and started choosing presence. I stopped measuring my worth in numbers and started measuring it in how often I treated myself with respect.

My why stopped being about "not getting worse" and became about living better right now, in this body, with this life.

Now, when the motivation fades or the self-doubt sneaks in, I remind myself:

I'm not chasing perfection.

I'm choosing consistency.

I'm not proving anything.

I'm remembering why I care.

Because real talk, your why doesn't have to be loud or impressive and it doesn't have to inspire anyone else. It just has to bring *you* back home to yourself.

That shift, from shame-driven to soul-driven, didn't miraculously make everything easy, but it made it feel *possible.*

And that's more than enough to keep going.

———

healing from setbacks without starting over

. . .

"You don't have to start over. You just have to keep going from where you are."

— Unknown

SETBACKS AREN'T the end of the story, they're part of it.

You don't experience them because you're weak, undisciplined, or broken, but because you're alive, and because life is unpredictable and messy, and sometimes diabetes doesn't care how well you planned. It just does its thing while you're juggling stress, hormones, family, work, exhaustion, emotions, and a body that occasionally acts like it's on its own schedule.

The idea that success means moving in a perfectly straight line? That's a myth sold by diet culture and productivity influencers. Real life looks more like a squiggly line drawn by a toddler on a sugar rush. But you know what? That line still moves forward.

You're not falling behind when you experience setbacks. You're navigating, and more importantly, you're learning the rhythm of resilience.

. . .

When One Slip Feels Like a Slide

Diet culture trains us to panic at the first wobble.

Miss a workout? "Might as well quit."

Eat dessert? "The day's ruined."

Have a tough week? "I've lost all my progress."

That kind of thinking convinces you that progress is fragile, and that one "bad" decision erases months of effort. But it's not true.

Progress isn't wiped away because of a few hard days. It's layered, built over time, and strengthened through repetition. Every step you've taken still counts and very effort still matters. Every comeback still builds something lasting.

You don't lose everything when life gets messy. You just lose your footing for a minute, and the good news? You can always find it again.

The Message Behind the Mess

Every setback carries information, not judgment. It's not your body trying to betray you, it's your body trying to communicate.

Sometimes the message is simple: you're exhausted. You need rest, not restriction. You need comfort, not control. Sometimes it's a sign your goals are too big, your plan too rigid, or your expectations are too high.

Setbacks show you where your systems need support. Treat them like feedback, instead of failure. And once you stop viewing them as verdicts, you can start using them as data to build something stronger and more sustainable.

Been There, Felt That

"I skipped one workout and ended up in a 'screw-it' spiral for three weeks. I didn't really want to quit, I just thought I had to go back to square one, and that felt defeating. Turns out, there is no square one. Just the next step forward."

Re-Entry, Not "Starting Over"

There was a time when I treated every detour like a disaster. I'd mess up once, panic, and start rewriting my whole plan. Now, I think of those moments as re-entry points.

When you're ready to step back in, skip the dramatics. You don't need a redemption arc. You just need honesty. "I had a rough week. Now I'm choosing to re-engage." That's it. No shame or guilt trip required.

Start with one small anchor habit that reconnects you to care without overwhelming you. It could be a glass of water before coffee, a quick blood-sugar check before lunch, or a slow walk after dinner. Do this not to punish yourself, but as a signal to yourself: I'm back. I'm still in this.

Then set an intention that feels gentle and real. Not "I'm going to crush it this week," but "I'm going to take care of myself today." That's enough.

And when resistance shows up, as it always does, don't fight it with guilt. Meet it with curiosity. "Why does this feel hard right now?" "What would make this 10% easier?" "How can I support myself instead of scolding myself?"

Re-entry isn't about being perfect. It's about showing yourself grace and giving yourself the permission to take the next imperfect step forward.

You Don't Have to Earn a Fresh Start

We've been conditioned to believe that recommitting to ourselves requires proof, and that we have to be "good" again for a few days before we deserve grace. But that's nonsense.

You don't need to check all the boxes before you're allowed to try again. You don't need to lose five pounds first or get your A1C back down to feel worthy. You are allowed to pick yourself up mid-mess and you are allowed to begin again at any moment.

There is no expiration date on effort.

Your wellness journey isn't a straight shot from broken to healed. It's a loop of progress, pause, setback, recommitment, and growth. It circles back on itself in different ways, each time with a little more wisdom, and a little more self-trust.

Some days, the loop is wide and you feel steady and confident. Other days, it tightens and causes you to trip, stumble, and forget what you're capable of. But every loop teaches you something. Every one brings you closer to the version of yourself that doesn't panic at a stumble.

Healing isn't about never falling. It's about falling softer, rising faster, and learning to trust that you can always begin again.

———

What Helped Me Most

I used to see setbacks as proof that I wasn't cut out for this. One bad day could unravel weeks of consistency. I'd fall into a shame spiral that took days, sometimes weeks, to crawl out of. It felt like I was constantly rebuilding from scratch.

But what finally helped me most was realizing that there is no "scratch." There is no reset button. Every effort, every small win, and every comeback still counted. Nothing was wasted.

I started celebrating what I called *re-entry days*, the days I chose to come back to myself. The morning I checked my blood sugar again after avoiding it for days, the night I made a balanced dinner instead of saying "screw it, or the walk I took just because I knew it would help me breathe. Those moments weren't restarts. They were reconnections.

Now, when I hit a rough patch, I don't try to fix everything at once. I start with one act of care: drink some water, stretch, check in, breathe. Each one is a brick in the foundation of my resilience.

And every single time I choose to return, no matter how messy or delayed, it strengthens the part of me that believes I can.

You don't have to start over. You just have to keep going from where you are.

That's not weakness. It's wisdom and growth. And that's how real healing happens: quietly, patiently, and one brave return at a time.

———

journaling
without eye rolls

. . .

"You don't have to write a love letter to your inner child under a full moon. Just get the thoughts out of your head."

— Unknown

WHEN SOMEONE SAYS "YOU SHOULD JOURNAL," half of us cringe a little. The word comes with baggage. It conjures up visions of aesthetic notebooks, gold pens, flawless handwriting, and long emotional entries that feel more performative than helpful.

Meanwhile, your real life looks more like this:

"Today sucked. I'm tired. Blood sugar is dumb. Diabetes is stupid. I need a nap. The end."

And you know what? That's just as valid friend.

You don't need to be poetic. You don't need to be deep. You don't even have to like writing. Journaling isn't about performing, it's about unloading the chaos in your head. It's about creating a place where you can get the mess out of your head and onto paper (or a screen) before it swallows your focus and your peace. Reflection isn't about being profound, but about getting unstuck.

. . .

What Journaling Actually Does

At its core, journaling is just noticing. It's noticing what's going well, what's frustrating, and what you keep repeating but wishing you wouldn't.

It's not homework, it's awareness.

When you put words to what's swirling around in your head, you can see your thoughts instead of drowning in them. It's how you catch yourself spiraling before you land face-first in the shame puddle. It's how you process emotions before they explode out sideways, and it's how you start connecting dots like, "Huh. Every time I skip lunch, my dinner turns into a free-for-all," or "My anxiety's worse when I don't sleep."

The act of noticing is the act of caring, and it says I'm paying attention to me.

Been There, Felt That

"I always thought journaling meant lighting a candle and pouring my soul out in cursive. Turns out, it can also mean scribbling 'this sucks' three times and closing the notebook. Still helps."

Why It Feels So Hard

Most of us resist journaling because it feels like another thing we're "supposed to" do perfectly. We think we need to have the right journal, the right mindset, and the right words. We think it's supposed to be deep or profound, or that we're supposed to end every entry with gratitude and a moral lesson.

But you don't need to write a Hallmark card to heal.

Some days your journal might be pages of insight. Other days, it's "I'm over it." Both matter. Three sentences are enough. One messy bullet point is enough. You can write in your phone, on a napkin, in the back of your planner, or not at all. Voice notes count too.

And yes, it can be scary to face what's in your head. But the truth is, putting your feelings on paper doesn't make them bigger. It makes them smaller. When you can see them, you can start to work with them instead of around them, or pretending they don't exist.

Make It Yours

There are no journaling police. There is no wrong way to do it. You can voice record your thoughts while driving to work, write on sticky notes and slap them on your mirror, or bullet list your entire day in chaos shorthand:

"Feeling meh. BG high. Need water. Craving tacos. Will deal later."

That's still reflection.

Start messy and stay messy if you want. The point isn't to create a masterpiece. It's to create space to pause, breathe, and listen to yourself for five minutes before the world gets loud again.

The Power of Journaling in Diabetes Care

Here's where journaling becomes quietly powerful. It doesn't just help you mentally, but it helps you manage your diabetes in a more compassionate, personal way.

When you jot down patterns or thoughts, you start noticing things data alone can't show you. You see how your mood, sleep, stress, food, and movement all dance together. You see how your numbers reflect your life, not your worth.

Journaling turns your care plan into a conversation instead of a command and gives you the words to advocate for yourself at appointments because you actually understand your own trends. It lets you celebrate the small wins that don't make it into your CGM graphs but matter just as much, like getting through a tough day without giving up on yourself.

You're not writing a diary, you're building a record of resilience.

When You Don't Know What to Write

If you're staring at a blank page wondering what to say, start with the simplest prompts:

- What do I need today that I'm not giving myself?
- What's actually working better than I realized?
- What triggered me recently, and what do I wish I'd done differently?
- Where am I showing more resilience than I give myself credit for?
- If my body could talk to me right now, what would it say?

You're not writing for an audience, you're writing to get closer to your truth.

———

What Helped Me Most

I used to think journaling was only for people who were already emotionally evolved or who had perfect handwriting and free mornings for meditation. That definitely wasn't me. But what I learned is that journaling doesn't have to be pretty, it just has to be honest.

Some of my most healing entries looked nothing like wisdom. They were rants, scribbles, and Notes app dumps at midnight. Sticky notes in my car that said "You're okay, keep going." Sometimes all I wrote was, "This blows." Sometimes I wrote one tiny win: "Didn't ignore my glucose monitor today." Sometimes I just wrote, "TRY AGAIN TOMORROW."

I learned it wasn't what I wrote that mattered, it was the act of writing it at all. It was showing up for myself when I didn't feel worth showing up for.

Journaling became my pressure valve and a place where I didn't have to fix, filter, or explain. It became the quiet space between mess and clarity, where I could look at my thoughts and choose which ones to keep.

And somewhere in that process, I started building something bigger than insight: self-trust. I learned to spot my own patterns without shame, and started treating my thoughts like data, not evidence against me. And I finally started listening to myself the way I'd listen to someone I love.

Now, on the days when my numbers suck, when motivation disappears on me again, or when life feels heavy, I don't try to "get it together." I grab a pen, dump the noise, and remind myself:

This isn't a confession.

It's a conversation.

And I'm still in it.

———

wrapping up part 2: mindset shifts and mental health

"You can't heal a body you constantly criticize or a life you refuse to participate in."

— Unknown

If you've made it through Part 2, take a second to let that sink in.

You've just done some of the hardest work there is, the inner work. The kind that doesn't show up in lab results or before-and-after photos. The kind that asks you to sit with uncomfortable truths, rewrite old stories, and finally start believing you're worth the effort it takes to heal.

This section wasn't about carbs or cardio. It was about the conversations you have with yourself when no one's watching, the ones that can either build you up or break you down. It's about the fear, the perfectionism, the comparison, the burnout, and the quiet moments when you wonder if all this effort is really worth it.

And through it all, you kept showing up, kept asking better questions, kept turning judgment into curiosity, shame into self-compassion, and chaos into awareness. That's mindset work and mental-health work. And it counts.

If Part 1 helped you *see yourself* beyond the diagnosis, Part 2 helped you *believe in yourself* beyond the struggle.

This journey isn't about learning to control everything. It's about learning to trust yourself in the process.

You don't need to be perfect to make progress.

You don't need motivation to matter.

You don't need to have it all figured out to start feeling better.

You just need to keep showing up with honesty, grace, and the tiniest bit of stubborn faith that you can grow through what you're going through.

————

What Helped Me Most

What helped me most in this season of mindset work wasn't a new routine or a breakthrough strategy. It was learning to pause and to notice when I was spiraling. It was questioning the voice that told me I was behind and to catch myself in old patterns and choose something gentler.

What helped me most was realizing that healing is not a straight line, it's a conversation. Some days, I had to talk myself into trying again. Other days, I surprised myself with how far I'd come. And the more I practiced listening instead of lecturing myself, the easier it got to stay in the game.

What helped me most was giving myself permission to be both the work in progress *and* the masterpiece at the same time. To celebrate the small wins and to stop waiting for motivation. I redefined "doing my best" as whatever was possible that day.

Because mindset work isn't a one-time shift. It's a lifelong practice of remembering who you are, even when the world (or your blood sugar) tries to convince you otherwise.

And if no one's told you this lately: you're doing the brave work. The real work. The kind that doesn't always feel glamorous, but changes your whole damn life in the long run.

————

Now, we move forward.

Part 3 is where it all starts coming together: the habits, the healing, and the everyday choices that turn awareness into action. It's where mindset meets momentum, and where you start living all the truths you've been collecting here.

So take what you've learned, breathe a little deeper, and step into this next part with curiosity and confidence.

Because this time, you're not just surviving, you're leading your own comeback story.

part three
habits, healing,
and everyday wins

"Success is the product of daily habits, not once-in-a-lifetime transformations."

— James Clear

This is where we shift from mindset to motion, from what's in your head to how you live it out.

But don't panic: this is *not* a part of the book where I suddenly tell you to wake up at 5 a.m., start drinking green smoothies, or count almonds for funsies.

This section is about building *realistic*, sustainable habits. Habits that work with your actual life, not against it, and ones that feel like a kindness to yourself, not a punishment for your diagnosis.

We're going to talk about things like how to stop labeling food as "good" or "bad," how to finally quit quitting, and how to set goals that don't make you want to disappear into a couch cushion. We'll unpack the subtle art of doing one thing at a time, moving your body without hating it, and finding the right people to walk alongside you (even if your real-life support system is…a lot).

This is the part where we remind ourselves: wellness isn't something you achieve and then keep forever. It's something you practice. It's the *showing up,* the *keep going,* and the small wins that don't get applause but matter more than we realize.

Ready to build something that lasts?

Let's go.

food is not a moral test

. . .

"When we make food the enemy, we lose the ability to listen to what our body is asking for."

— Christy Harrison, MPH, RD

LET'S talk about one of the biggest mind games in diabetes care: food.

Not just food as fuel or food as comfort, but food as a daily report card. Food as guilt, and as the thing you're expected to manage flawlessly while the world watches and comments.

If you've ever stared at your plate and thought, *"I shouldn't eat that,"* or felt like you failed because of something you ate, then you already know what food judgment feels like. But here's the truth: Food is not good or bad, and you are not good or bad because of what you eat. Food is just food, and your worth is not based on what's on your plate.

How We Got Here

For people with type 2 diabetes, food doesn't just nourish the body, it becomes the battleground. We're given handouts with pie charts and told to "watch our carbs." We're bombarded with conflicting advice, and somewhere in the middle of it all, we start believing that the way we eat defines our character.

We've been told we lack discipline, and that we should "know better." And if we really cared, we'd skip the cake, count the macros, and never, ever mess up.

And little by little, that kind of talk drowns out something essential: our own instincts. The body's quiet cues about hunger, satisfaction, and comfort get replaced by fear, rules, and shame. And before long, every bite feels like a test you're destined to fail.

Been There, Felt That

"There was a stretch of time when I couldn't eat a piece of bread without hearing a voice in my head whisper, 'You're ruining every-thing.' I wasn't just counting carbs, it was like I was counting failures. It took years to realize the fear wasn't about the food, but about what I thought eating it said about me."

You Don't Have to Earn Your Carbs

Carbs are not evil and sugar is not the enemy. You are not required to justify your choices to anyone, not to your doctor, your family, or that internal critic narrating your every move.

There's a difference between mindful eating and micromanaged eating.

Mindful eating asks, *"How does this make me feel?"*

Micromanaged eating demands, *"Do I deserve this?"*

The first leads to awareness while the second leads to exhaustion.

When we stop labeling food as "good" or "bad," we can finally start noticing what our bodies have been trying to tell us all along: that eating isn't a performance, it's a relationship. And like any relation-ship, it requires trust, curiosity, and communication, not judgment.

Trusting yourself around food doesn't happen overnight. It's a process of unlearning and of paying attention instead of policing yourself.

It starts with simple shifts: checking in before you eat instead of checking out afterward, noticing how food makes you feel rather than how it makes you look. Asking, *"Am I hungry, or am I trying to soothe something else?"* and answering honestly without punishment.

When you get curious, the guilt starts to lose its grip, and you begin to see that overeating, restricting, or craving aren't signs of weakness, they're signals. And every signal is a chance to learn.

This Isn't About "Letting Yourself Go"

One of the biggest fears people have when they stop following strict food rules is that everything will fall apart, and that if they let go of control, they'll lose control.

But if you're honest, hasn't the control game already made you miserable?

Most people don't struggle because they gave themselves too much permission, but because they've been trapped in cycles of shame, restriction, and rebellion for years. And the truth is, judgment doesn't create consistency. Compassion does.

When you remove the shame, you make space for intention. When you remove the rules, you make room for rhythm, because permission isn't the enemy, it's the beginning of peace.

Instead of, *"Should I eat this?"* try asking, *"What does support look like for me right now?"*

Sometimes support looks like a balanced plate that steadies your energy, and sometimes it looks like eating the cupcake at your kid's birthday party and being fully present for the laughter instead of mentally tallying carbs.

Sometimes it looks like grabbing a snack before you crash because your body is whispering, *please don't ignore me again.*

You don't have to analyze every decision. But you *do* have to care enough to stay connected and to begin to eat with awareness instead of anxiety.

. . .

You're Not Failing. You're Learning.

If you've ever woken up after a "bad food day" and vowed to make up for it by being extra strict, you're not alone. But guilt isn't a plan. It's you beating yourself up and calling it accountability.

Real growth happens when you move from control to care. When you shift from "How do I fix this?" to "How do I support myself better next time?"

That shift isn't glamorous, and it's not instant, but it's how you build a relationship with food that feels calm, instead of chaotic.

Because the goal isn't perfection, it's peace.

––––––––

What Helped Me Most

One of the biggest turning points for me was when I stopped treating food like a moral test and started using it as feedback.

Instead of labeling meals as good or bad, I began asking, *How did that make me feel, physically and emotionally? Did I eat in a rush, or did I actually taste it? Was I trying to cope, or to nourish?*

And when I realized that guilt had become my default coping mechanism, I decided to try something radical: I let myself eat a cookie without a lecture. I didn't "earn" it, I didn't make up for it later, I just enjoyed it and moved on.

It sounds small, but it cracked something open in me. That single act of grace reminded me that trust isn't built in grand gestures but in the quiet moments when you choose honesty over punishment.

Now, when I catch myself thinking, *"I was bad today,"* I stop and reframe it: *"That didn't work for me. What can I do differently next time?"*

That one reframe gave me my power back. It turned guilt into growth, food into feedback, and meals into moments of connection instead of conflict.

Because when you can trust yourself at the table, you start trusting yourself everywhere else, too.

––––––––

your plate, your plan

. . .

"The best diet is the one you can live with, not the one you have to suffer through."

— Unknown

IF YOU'VE BEEN LIVING with type 2 diabetes for more than five minutes, you've probably been hit with a buffet of conflicting advice:

"Go low carb."

"Keto cured my uncle."

"You just need to cut out sugar."

"Have you tried intermittent fasting?"

"No fruit. Ever."

Sound familiar?

Here's the deal: there is no one-size-fits-all way to eat for diabetes.

If there were, this book would be a pamphlet, and you'd already feel amazing.

But most of us were taught to follow someone else's rules, to ignore our own hunger cues, and to treat food like it's either medicine or poison. And that's not health, that's a truck load of stress with a side-car of shame.

So, instead of chasing the "perfect" diet, let's talk about building an approach that actually fits *you*.

Been There, Felt That

"I spent years jumping from one diet to the next: low carb, no carb, carnivore, keto, you name it. Every plan worked until it didn't. I finally realized I didn't need another rulebook, I needed a way of eating that respected both my blood sugar and my reality."

What Works for You Is What Matters

Managing diabetes through food isn't about perfection, it's about patterns. It's about learning what fuels you, what drains you, and what feels sustainable.

Your plate should support your life, not shrink it. It should stabilize your blood sugar most of the time, give you energy that lasts, work with your medications instead of against them, and, most importantly, include foods you actually enjoy.

If your "healthy eating" plan leaves you hungry, cranky, or afraid of social situations, that's not a healthy plan. That's a red flag in meal-plan form.

Because any plan that sacrifices your peace of mind to get your numbers "perfect" will eventually backfire, and you can't hate yourself into consistency.

So...What Should You Eat?

Here's the annoying but freeing answer: it depends.

Yes, there are general principles that help most people with diabetes like adding protein and fiber to slow blood sugar spikes, keeping meals balanced, staying hydrated, and paying attention to carb quality rather than just quantity.

But the details? Those belong to you.

What foods give *you* energy?

What meals fit your schedule, your culture, and your budget?

How does your body actually respond? Not what an influencer's body does, but yours?

The plan that works is the one that makes room for your real life, the one you can stick to when work's chaotic, your kid's got practice, and dinner happens in the car.

How to Tell When It's Working

Your eating plan is working when you feel like you're living, not just surviving. It's working when your blood sugar is more stable, but your mental energy is too, when you feel nourished, not deprived, and when food becomes a source of confidence, instead of confusion.

It's working when you can eat dinner without mentally calculating what you have to "make up for" tomorrow, when you stop describing your day as "good" or "bad" based on a number, and when you start trusting yourself to make adjustments without guilt.

If you're constantly rebounding or restarting, it doesn't mean you lack discipline, it means your plan lacks flexibility.

Be cautious of any eating plan that thrives on extremes.

If it bans entire food groups, promises a "cure," shames your cravings, or convinces you your culture's foods are the problem, it's not helping.

If you're following advice from someone who doesn't live in your body, take it lightly, and if a diet makes you feel like you're failing every time you're imperfect, it's time to ditch that plan.

Nutrition should empower you, not exhaust you.

Building a Real-Life Plate

You don't need to measure every gram or memorize a macro chart. You just need a sense of balance that works for your day-to-day life.

Maybe that means filling half your plate with veggies, a quarter with lean protein, and a quarter with complex carbs. Maybe it means cutting your rice portion in half and adding beans or avocado for fiber and fat. Maybe it means not skipping breakfast because you finally realized starting your day hungry sets you up to crash later.

There's no perfect plate, only one that supports how you want to feel.

This is not about deprivation. It's about creating meals that give you energy, stability, and peace, and about learning what "enough" feels like, both physically and emotionally.

It's about finding joy again in eating, because you deserve that, too.

———

What Helped Me Most

What helped me most was realizing that I didn't need another strict plan, I needed permission to listen to my body.

For years, I lived in diet mode, jumping from low-carb to "clean eating" to fasting to whatever was trending on Instagram that week. I confused control with success. I believed if it wasn't hard, it wasn't working.

But the truth was, all that control disconnected me from the one thing I actually needed: awareness.

When I finally slowed down and paid attention, not to calories or points, but to patterns, things started to make a lot more sense. I noticed which meals gave me steady energy, which left me sluggish, and which kept my blood sugar balanced without leaving me miserable.

I stopped labeling days as "good" or "bad" and started asking one question: *Did what I ate help me feel how I want to feel today?*

I stopped trying to master someone else's plan and started building my own. I constructed a plan that could survive holidays, stress, travel, and real life, and one that didn't punish me for being a literal human being.

Now, I eat with intention, not obsession. I track my progress through how I feel, instead of how "perfect" my meals look.

Because food isn't supposed to make you anxious, it's supposed to help you live.

So if you've been chasing the perfect diet, here's your permission to stop. You don't need a plan that impresses anyone else.

You need one that makes you feel at home in your own body again.

———

diet culture detox

. . .

"Diet culture is the most socially accepted form of disordered thinking."

— Christy Harrison

THIS ISN'T JUST A DETOX.

It's a rebellion against the system that taught us to hate ourselves in the name of health.

Diet culture shows up wearing confidence and control like designer labels. It promises transformation, validation, and a sense of order in a world that feels messy. It tells you that if you could just be smaller, stricter, stronger, or more disciplined you'd finally feel free.

But what it actually delivers?

Guilt.

Exhaustion.

And a lifetime subscription to never feeling good enough.

And when you're living with type 2 diabetes, that noise gets even louder. Because now it's not just about what you eat, it's about whether you're "doing it right," whether you're a "good diabetic," and whether you've "earned" your numbers or your doctor's approval. As if health were a report card instead of a relationship with your body.

But here's the truth:

You don't owe the world a smaller, more disciplined version of yourself to prove your worth.

Been There, Felt That

"I used to think every craving was a test, and every bite of cake was a failure. I didn't even enjoy food anymore. I just calculated it, feared it, and felt guilty about it. That wasn't wellness. It was war. I was so focused on being 'good' that I forgot to be human."

What Diet Culture Really Is

Diet culture isn't just a set of food rules, it's a belief system that moralizes your body and your choices. It says thin is good, hunger is weakness, control is virtue, and failure is inevitable. It turns food into math formulas, movement into punishment, and self-worth into a daily negotiation.

You've seen it. You've most likely lived it, too. Maybe it sounds like this:

You skip dinner and call it discipline. You eat something you love and call it guilt. You compare your plate, your body, and your numbers because someone somewhere told you that perfection is the price of health. No pain, no gain.

And when you have diabetes, that voice has a megaphone.

Suddenly, every carb feels like a confession of guilt and every medication refill feels like proof you've failed.

But you haven't failed.

You've just been operating under a system that profits off your self-doubt.

•   •   •

Unlearning the Lies

Unlearning diet culture isn't about giving up on health, it's about reminding yourself what health actually means.

It's separating your worth from your weight, and it's feeding your body because it deserves energy, not because you're trying to fix it.

It's about acknowledging that discipline without compassion isn't "being strong", it's self-punishment.

Start by noticing the little moments when diet culture sneaks in.

That tiny wince when you see a higher number on the scale.

The mental apology when you eat something "off plan."

The guilt when you rest instead of pushing through.

Those are not facts. They're learned reactions, and guess what?

You can unlearn them.

The work is simple, but it's not easy. It looks like asking better questions:

- What would self-respect look like right now?
- Who gave me this rule and does it still serve me?
- If my best friend said this about themselves, what would I say back?

Each time you pause and question instead of obeying, you chip away at the old script.

And eventually, you start writing a new one.

Diet culture doesn't just shape how you eat, it also shapes how you *think* about yourself.

It tells you that joy must be earned, that rest must be justified, and that you're only as good as your last "good day."

But healing means rejecting all of that.

It means saying things like:

I'm not cheating, I'm eating.

My blood sugar is a number, not a judgment.

I don't have to earn my worth by restricting my joy.

When you start to live that truth, food stops being a battlefield, and instead it becomes what it was always meant to be: connection, energy, nourishment, and sometimes comfort.

And that's freedom, not failure.

Been There, Felt That (Part Two)

"I once went six months without eating a single bite of bread. When I finally did, I exhaled with such relief because I realized I had spent half a year at war with myself for no reason. That first sandwich wasn't weakness or failure or falling of the wagon. It was finally coming to a truce with carbs."

What Helped Me Most

There came a point when I realized that diet culture wasn't helping me "stay accountable", it was keeping me stuck.

I'd been measuring good days by how little I ate, how compliant I looked, and how well I could pretend I didn't miss the foods I loved.

And honestly? I was miserable.

What helped me most was finally questioning the entire system.

Who decided that hunger was failure?

Who decided that thinness equals health?

And who decided that I should feel guilty for eating fruit?

Once I realized I didn't believe those rules anymore, I stopped living by them.

I started asking, "Does this food serve me right now?" instead of, "Is this food allowed?"

Sometimes the answer was yes, and sometimes it was no. But more importantly, I started making those decisions without shame.

And that calm, grounded, unapologetic choice felt powerful.

I stopped treating food like a test I could fail, stopped worshipping willpower, and started practicing putting trust in myself.

I learned that nourishment doesn't have to hurt or be earned. It just has to support you.

These days, I don't chase "good" days anymore. I chase peaceful ones.

That looks like eating what feels right, moving because it feels good, and treating my body like an ally instead of an obstacle to overcome.

Because real, total wellness isn't about control, it's about connection to your body, to your needs, and to your life.

And when you finally make peace with food, you make space for everything else you were too busy hating yourself to enjoy.

———

accountability, not isolation

. . .

"You can do it alone, but you don't have to. And honestly? It's a lot harder that way."

— Unknown

LET'S get one thing straight: You don't have to do this alone.

And honestly? You were never meant to.

We love our independence, especially when we've spent years managing something like type 2 diabetes. Independence feels safe, predictable, and controlled. It's how we survive the noise of everyone else's advice and opinions.

We say things like:

"I know what to do. I just need to do it."

"I don't want to burden anyone."

"I'm fine on my own."

But beneath that independence, there's often burnout, quiet exhaustion, and the fear that if we *do* let people in and then struggle anyway, they'll think we're weak, unmotivated, or incapable.

Been There, Felt That

"I used to say I didn't need anyone. I had my to-do lists, my podcasts, my Pinterest boards full of motivation and meal plans. But somehow, I kept quitting on myself. Turns out, the missing piece wasn't more discipline, it was finding people who wouldn't let me disappear when it got hard."

What Accountability Actually Looks Like

Real accountability isn't a boot camp instructor barking orders, a spreadsheet, a stopwatch, or a guilt trip disguised as support.

It's personal, honest, and it's messy.

It's someone saying,

"Hey, you haven't checked in lately. You okay?"

It's the friend who texts,

"Let's take a walk, even if you don't feel like it."

It's a gentle voice that reminds you why you started when your inner critic is screaming, *What's the point?*

True accountability isn't about being monitored, it's about being *met right where you're at.* It's about being seen in the middle of the struggle and reminded that trying again still counts.

It's someone who doesn't flinch at your frustration or your setbacks, who doesn't need you to be "good" to be worth supporting, and who simply says, "You're not alone in this. Let's keep going."

That's what real accountability feels like: support without shame, encouragement without perfectionism, and compassion without pity.

But What If You're Not a "Group" Person?

Not everyone thrives in big communities or public check-ins. That's okay. Accountability doesn't have to be loud to be powerful.

It can look like a single friend who knows when to nudge you.

A journal where you track your goals honestly.

A calendar reminder that says, "Hey, you promised yourself you'd move today."

Even your dog giving you side-eye when you skip your walk counts as accountability some days.

It's not about the method. It's about finding that connection that resonates with you.

Maybe it's your sister who knows when you're struggling before you admit it.

Maybe it's a mentor who checks in after a hard week.

Maybe it's an online community where people just *get it*, no explanation needed.

You don't have to share everything, but you do need to share *something*.

Because silence breeds isolation, and isolation feeds the lie that you're the only one who finds this hard.

You're not.

Isolation can feel easier at first. There's no pressure, no eyes on you, and no one to disappoint.

But here's what really happens when you isolate:

You start living in your own head and the thoughts in there aren't always kind.

"Everyone else is doing better."

"Why can't I get it together?"

"Maybe I'm just not cut out for this."

Sound familiar?

That's not self-discipline, it's self-sabotage dressed as independence.

Community interrupts those spirals. It replaces comparison with connection, normalizes the messy middle, and turns shame into shared strength.

You don't need a crowd cheering you on every day. You just need one person who believes in your next step when you can't see it yourself.

Somewhere along the way, we confused accountability with surveillance.

But the kind of accountability that actually changes lives doesn't come from someone keeping tabs, but from someone keeping space.

Accountability isn't someone standing over you with a clipboard; it's someone standing beside you when you want to give up.

It's not about judgment or pressure. It's about belonging and partnership.

You don't need a coach or a community to *make* you do the work. You need one that reminds you *why* it's worth doing.

What Helped Me Most

For years, I wore "I've got this" like a badge of honor. I thought needing help meant I wasn't committed enough, strong enough, or serious enough.

So I did it all alone. And it worked for a while…until it didn't.

Eventually, isolation caught up with me. I wasn't failing because I didn't know what to do. I was failing because I was so tired of doing it alone. I realized I needed a lifeline.

The turning point came when I finally let someone in. I didn't join a group right away, or get a new plan. I just found myself one trusted person who saw me trying and didn't turn away when I stumbled. They didn't lecture me, or try to fix me. They simply said, "You're allowed to need people."

I started small with sending a text after a hard appointment instead of pretending I was fine.

I'll be honest, the first time I joined an online community, I hated it. Everyone was so mean to each other. I knew immediately it wasn't the place for me. I needed a space where I left feeling more empowered than when I arrived, a space that lifted me up when I felt like I was slowly slipping under the water, a space where I heard a chorus of people singing the same tune as me. That's when Sugar Mama Strong Diabetes Support for Women was born and I finally found my people. Not only did I start sharing my numbers regularly, I started posting small wins instead of hiding until I had something "big" to celebrate. Replying "me too" when someone else was struggling instead of scrolling past it helped me connect with others who were in the same boat.

Those moments taught me something I wish I'd learned sooner: connection doesn't drain your strength, it compounds it.

Now, I build accountability into my health plan on purpose. Not as a safety net, but as a foundation. Because support isn't a backup strategy, it's an integral part of the solution.

And the more I let people show up for me, the more I found myself showing up for *me*, too.

So if you've been white-knuckling this journey alone, here's your permission to loosen your grip.

You can do it solo, sure, but you don't have to.

Let someone in.

Because accountability doesn't make you weak, it makes you *seen*. And being seen might be just the thing that saves you from quitting one more time.

Accountability reminds you that you don't have to disappear when things get hard. But not all support feels the same, and learning who belongs in your corner is just as important as letting someone in.

———

support systems: building a circle that holds you up

. . .

"Sometimes the bravest thing you can do is ask for help and let yourself receive it."

— Brené Brown

LET'S JUST SAY IT: Support systems can make or break your wellness journey.

When they're strong, they hold you up like scaffolding. They're steady, sturdy, and exactly what keeps you from collapsing when life gets heavy.

When they're shaky, or missing altogether, it feels like trying to climb a mountain with a backpack full of bricks and no one to pass you the water bottle.

And when you've spent most of your life being praised for your independence, when you've been told to "handle it," to "be strong," or to "not make a fuss", asking for help can feel like failure.

But the truth is, needing people doesn't make you fragile. It makes you like everyone else.

Been There, Felt That

"For a long time, I believed support was something other people had. I figured I needed to tough it out, keep my head down, and deal with the highs and lows quietly because no one around me really understood the mental load of all this. Then I found one person who genuinely did, who didn't minimize it, didn't judge it, and didn't try to 'fix' it. Just understood. And that one connection made everything feel a little less heavy and a lot more possible."

Why You Can't (and Shouldn't) Do This Alone

Living with type 2 diabetes isn't a checklist, but a constant balancing act.

It's food, meds, movement, sleep, stress, emotions, appointments, numbers, guilt, and grace all woven into the same day. It's being your own health manager, cheerleader, and crisis response team, often before your morning coffee.

That's a lot for one person.

You weren't meant to carry it all alone.

You deserve people who hold space for all of it, the practical and the emotional, the messy and the miraculous. People who:

- Don't flinch when you say, "My blood sugar's tanking."
- Remind you that needing medication doesn't mean you've failed.
- Talk you off the ledge when your A1C isn't what you hoped.
- Celebrate the small wins you're too tired to notice.

Support doesn't have to be perfect, but it does have to be *present*.

Finding Your People (Without the Drama)

Here's the thing no one tells you: not everyone in your life will know how to support you and that's okay.

Some will love you deeply but not understand a thing about your diabetes.

Some will mean well but say the worst possible thing.

And some will get it, because they're walking the same road. And those people? They're gold.

Your job is to build your circle *on purpose.*

Look for people who listen more than they lecture, who validate instead of fixing, who ask what you need instead of assuming, and who leave you feeling lighter, not smaller.

And remember support doesn't always come from the people you've known the longest.

It can come from a friend you met online, a workout partner who became a confidant, or a community that finally makes you feel seen instead of "other."

Maybe your person is a spouse who learns your carb ratios, a friend who walks with you after dinner, or an online group that understands exactly what "sensor burnout" feels like.

The who matters less than the *how.*

What matters is that they see you and that they stay.

Real support is about holding, not about fixing. It's someone sitting beside you while you vent about your week, then saying, "You're doing better than you think."

It's the friend who checks in, because they care, not because they want updates. It's the message that says, "I know today's hard, but I'm proud of you for showing up anyway."

It's small moments, repeated often.

The text that says, "Drink your water."

The call that starts with, "Walk with me while we talk."

The eye contact that says, "You're safe here."

That's what real support feels like. It's not pressure, pity, or performance, just partnership.

And sometimes, real support also means accountability.

Someone who says, "You're allowed to rest, but I also know you'll feel better if you move."

Someone who calls you out *with love,* not judgment.

Support is knowing you don't have to face the hard days alone.

It's Okay to Outgrow People

Here's the hard part: not everyone can stay.

Some people won't meet you where you're going, some will minimize your diagnosis or mock your efforts, and some will disappear when you take the mask off and stop pretending everything's fine.

And that's painful.

But the reality is, you can love people from a distance.

You can forgive them without re-inviting their energy, and you can grieve what you hoped the relationship would be and still choose peace.

Outgrowing people doesn't mean you're cruel. It just means you're done shrinking to stay connected. And that my friend, is growth.

Protecting your peace is part of your health plan, too.

———

What Helped Me Most

When I first started focusing on my health, I thought I had to *earn* support.

I believed I needed to prove I was serious, prove I was "doing enough," and prove I wasn't going to be a burden.

But what helped me most was realizing that connection isn't a *reward*, but a *requirement*.

I started small. I told one person, "This is hard for me."

They didn't try to fix it. They just said, "Thanks for sharing with me. I'm here."

That opened the door for me. From there, I found spaces that felt safe and people who didn't need me to perform wellness, only live it.

In support groups, coaching calls, and everyday conversations, I started to see how many of us were quietly carrying the same weight. And hearing "me too" was so comforting.

I also learned that asking for help isn't the same as giving up.

It's actually a form of strength, a declaration that you want better, and you're willing to receive it.

Some days, support looked like someone bringing me dinner when

I was too exhausted to cook, and other days, it looked like my community reminding me, "Rest is still progress."

And slowly, I built a circle. My circle doesn't consist of perfect people, but *present* ones. The kind of people who don't just hold me accountable, but hold me up.

If you're reading this and thinking, "I don't have that," I want you to hear me: you can build it.

It might take time. It might mean widening your circle instead of clinging to what's familiar.

But you deserve support that feels steady, not conditional.

The right people won't make you feel like a burden for having needs.

They'll make you feel grounded, seen, and less alone.

And that kind of support doesn't just feel good in the moment.

It's what helps change last.

———

when support systems suck

. . .

"Just because someone loves you doesn't mean they know how to support you."

— Nakeia Homer

LET'S just get the hard truth out of the way: Not everyone is going to get it, and not everyone is going to be helpful. I know, ouch.

And sometimes, the people you love most, the ones you assumed would show up, don't.

Sometimes they minimize your needs, make jokes at your expense, roll their eyes when you say "no thanks" to dessert, and tell you to "just lose weight" like it's some sort of five-minute fix.

They treat your diagnosis like something you caused instead of something you're managing.

And honestly? It stings.

Because it's not coming from strangers, it's coming from *your* people. Family. Friends. Coworkers. The ones you hoped would have your back.

Been There, Felt That

"I kept hoping they'd get it, kept hoping someone would ask how I was really doing. But they never did. Eventually, I stopped waiting and started building the kind of support I actually needed."

When Love Comes with Side-Eye

Here's the part no one prepares you for: sometimes, taking care of yourself creates tension.

You'll set some boundaries. You'll skip the extra drink, say no to certain foods, or leave early to rest, and someone will act like you've declared war on fun.

You'll hear, "Just this once won't kill you," or "Don't be so dramatic," or my personal favorite, "You used to be more fun."

And that hurts. Because they're not seeing your effort as courage, they're seeing it as inconvenience for *them*.

But here's the truth hiding underneath all that noise: your growth is disrupting the status quo. When you start showing up differently: clearer, calmer, and more intentional, it shines a light on other people's comfort zones. And sometimes, they'll squint at the brightness.

You are allowed to grow anyway. And you're allowed to protect your peace, even if it makes other people uncomfortable.

You are not required to shrink or abandon your journey so others can stay the same.

What to Say When They Don't Understand

You don't owe anyone a PowerPoint presentation about your health, and you don't need to explain your glucose levels, your carb choices, or your treatment plan at every dinner table.

But it helps to have a few boundary-keeping phrases ready for those awkward moments:

- "I'm doing what works for me."
- "My health isn't up for discussion today."

• "I know you care, but this is what caring for myself looks like right now."

And sometimes, you don't need to say anything at all. A smile, a sip of water, and a quick subject change can say plenty.

Because real talk: You don't need anyone's permission to take care of yourself. Period. End of story.

Grieving the Support You Didn't Get

This part is hard, but we have to talk about it: Sometimes the people you counted on will let you down.

They'll dismiss your diagnosis, brush off your boundaries, and offer advice when what you really needed was empathy.

And you'll find yourself sitting with that mix of sadness, anger, and disappointment that you didn't see coming. That's a type of grief, and it's real, raw, and quiet.

You're grieving the version of the relationship you thought you had. You're mourning the expectation that someone would show up for you the way you've shown up for them. And that hurts.

Being honest and acknowledging that pain doesn't make you weak. The fact is, you can love people and still accept their limitations. You can try to understand their perspective and still protect your peace.

You can absolutely stop chasing the apology that may never come and start building the safety you deserve somewhere else.

Building the Support You Choose

If your current circle doesn't get it, build a new one. And know this: doing that doesn't make you disloyal, it's one of the healthiest things you can do for yourself.

Find spaces where you don't have to explain the basics.

Find people who don't wince when you talk about your A1C, who celebrate your wins, and who offer empathy instead of advice.

That might mean joining an online diabetes community, working with a coach, or connecting with one friend who just gets it.

Chosen family, internet friends, and wellness groups aren't second-best. They're proof that you can rebuild support from scratch.

You don't need the whole world to understand you. You just need a few people who say:

"Me too."

"You're not overreacting."

"I'm proud of you."

"Let's keep going."

Those voices? They'll get you through the hardest days.

———

What Helped Me Most

What helped me most was realizing that being disappointed by someone didn't mean I was asking for too much, it just meant I was probably asking the wrong person.

For a long time, I thought love and understanding came as a package deal. But the truth is, some people love you deeply and still can't meet you where you are, and that's not your failure. That's their limitation.

I had to stop measuring relationships by longevity and start measuring them by how they made me feel when I was vulnerable. Some connections strengthened when I got honest, and others faded. Both were information.

I also learned that I didn't need to keep handing out grace to people who weren't handling it with care. Protecting my peace was about my survival, not me being selfish.

Eventually, I stopped waiting for people to "come around" and started surrounding myself with people who were already ready. The ones who didn't need to understand every medical detail to say, "I'm here." People who believed me the first time I said I was tired.

Surrounding myself with those people didn't make all the hard moments disappear, but they helped me realize I wasn't walking through them alone anymore. And that made the tough times feel a bit easier.

If your support system isn't showing up, take that as your sign to build one that will.

Because here's the hard truth.

If someone makes you feel small for needing help, they're not part of your healing.

The people who truly get it won't shame you for struggling or rush you to be "better."

They'll meet you where you are or step aside.

And choosing distance from what hurts you?

That's not failure. That's self-respect.

———

why you keep quitting and how to quit that

. . .

"Success is the ability to go from failure to failure without losing your enthusiasm."

— Winston Churchill

LET'S cut to the chase: if you're sick of starting over, you're not alone and there's nothing wrong with you. You're just stuck in a loop that so many of us fall into: believing that if we're not perfect, we've failed.

And perfection? She's a sneaky little liar. She shows up dressed like discipline but secretly thrives on shame. She whispers:

"You already messed up. Might as well start Monday."

"This isn't the right time. Wait until life calms down."

"You'll never stick with it anyway, so why bother?"

Sound familiar?

Here's the thing: You don't need a new plan. You need a new pattern. Your plan isn't broken, it's your belief about "messing up" that is.

Why We Keep Quitting

Quitting rarely comes from laziness. It usually comes from exhaustion, pressure, or pain dressed as self-protection.

We quit because we're tired of trying so hard and feeling like it's never enough, because we're scared of failing publicly (again), and because it feels safer to stop than to risk another disappointment.

And most of the time, we don't quit in a big dramatic way. There's no final speech or slammed notebook. We just...drift.

We miss a workout, or skip a check in, or avoid a doctor's appointment, or put the meter away "for a few days."

And before we know it, we've quietly ghosted our own goals.

But here's what matters most: you're not actually starting from scratch when you come back. Every single attempt leaves breadcrumbs of experience. You bring back insight, awareness, and resilience that didn't exist the first time.

You're not starting over, friend. You're starting again, from wisdom. And that's progress.

Been There, Felt That

"I was doing everything right until I missed a workout, ate a whole sleeve of Oreos, and suddenly decided the whole week was a waste. So I quit. Again. But this time I lied and told myself I was just 'taking a break.' That break ended up lasting six months."

How to Quit Quitting

You're not someone who "can't stick with things." You're someone who's been surviving in a system that worships extremes and you've been told that discipline is everything and compassion is weakness. That if you struggle, it means you don't want it badly enough. But that's not truth, that's the conditioning we've been fed for decades.

So here's how we rewrite it.

Start with baby steps that actually fit your life. Consistency isn't about intensity, it's about sustainability. A ten-minute walk counts.

Taking your meds counts. Drinking water counts. One mindful choice adds up faster than one perfect week followed by burnout.

When that shame voice pops up and says "you failed again", talk back to it. Out loud if you have to.

Say: *"I didn't fail. I paused. And I get to begin again."*

Then plan for setbacks. Not *if* they happen, *when* they happen. Because they will. But a setback doesn't have to become a spiral.

Your new mantra: *"One rough day doesn't erase all the good ones."*

And finally, keep showing up, especially when you don't feel like it. Motivation will flake, energy will dip, and life will throw curveballs. But tiny, doable, unglamorous action creates momentum. And momentum builds trust that becomes the thing that keeps you going long after motivation has left the building.

The next time you want to quit, *don't.*

Pause.

Rest.

Cry in your car if you need to.

Take a breath, eat the cookie, or text a friend who gets it.

Then, when you can, take one small action that reconnects you to yourself.

Check your blood sugar, go for a short walk, drink some water, and remind yourself that you are not the same person who quit last time. You're someone who's learning how to stay.

And that, my friend, is growth in its rawest, realest form.

————

What Helped Me Most

I used to think quitting was my flaw. That if I could just find the "right" plan, I'd finally be fixed. But what I eventually learned was that my real problem wasn't quitting, but how I defined success.

I thought success meant perfection. No skipped workouts or off-plan meals or bad numbers. So every time I missed a mark, I treated it like failure instead of feedback, and that constant pressure made me want to disappear.

Perspective changed when I started building permission into my plan. I gave myself permission to rest, to stumble, and to show up messy instead of not at all.

I created what I call my *"life-is-lifing plan."* On the good days, it's movement, meal prep, journaling, the whole deal. On the hard days, it might just be checking my blood sugar once, drinking a glass of water, and sending one honest text: *"Today sucks."* Both versions count and both keep me connected to my goals.

I also stopped making dramatic "day-one" declarations. I didn't need to restart my life, I just needed to re-enter it, quietly, kindly, and one small choice at a time.

Now when I feel myself slipping, I ask one question: *"What's the next right thing I can do for myself?"* Sometimes the answer is movement, sometimes it's rest, but either way, I feel more grounded when I refocus myself instead of bailing on the journey completely. Because what helped me most wasn't willpower. It was giving myself enough grace to be imperfect and still keep going.

You don't have to wait to feel ready and you don't have to do it all perfectly. You just have to keep the door open between where you are and where you want to go.

That's not quitting. It's becoming.

———

goal setting that doesn't suck

. . .

"You don't need bigger goals. You need goals that make you feel safe enough to keep showing up."

— Dr. Sasha Heinz

LET'S talk about real goal setting. You know, the kind that doesn't make you want to throw your planner across the room.

If you've lived with type 2 diabetes for a while, you've probably been told to set SMART goals, track everything, and "stay consistent." Sounds simple enough, right? Except life isn't simple. It's unpredictable and chaotic, and when your blood sugar, emotions, and schedule all have minds of their own, those shiny goals can start to feel like traps.

We've all had that moment of motivation where we grab a notebook and decide, *This time it's going to be different.*

We write down things like:

"Lose 30 pounds."

"Work out 6 days a week."

"Never eat sugar again."

And for a few days, we're on fire…until life shows up. A stressful week, a missed workout, a craving, or a curveball. Suddenly, we feel like we're back at square one, calling ourselves inconsistent or undisciplined.

But here's the truth: you're not the problem. The problem is the goals themselves.

Big, dramatic goals sound exciting. But in the real world, where you're balancing blood sugar checks, work, relationships, and sleep deprivation, they're not sustainable. You don't need bigger goals, you need goals that fit your actual life.

Big goals are seductive because they promise transformation.

They make you feel powerful, capable, in control until they don't.

When your energy dips or your week goes sideways, those same goals can turn into proof that you've failed.

You didn't fail because you're lazy or uncommitted, but because your goals depended on perfection, and well, perfection doesn't exist in real life.

True success isn't built in the big moments. It's built in the small, quiet ones you show up even when you're tired, and when you make the next right choice instead of the "perfect" one.

When your goals make space for imperfection, you stop quitting every time things get hard, and you stop living in the land of all-or-nothing and start building consistency that actually lasts.

Been There, Felt That

"I used to set these massive goals that looked great on paper, like lose 50 pounds, meal prep every Sunday, or hit 10K steps every day. By week two, I was exhausted, behind, and drowning in guilt because real life kept getting in the way. I didn't fail because I lacked motivation. I failed because the goals didn't fit my life."

What Makes a Goal Work

Here's the thing: good goals aren't heroic, they're honest.

They don't ask you to become someone else overnight. Instead they meet you exactly where you are and move with you as life shifts.

A goal that actually works does three things: it bends instead of breaks, it builds self-trust instead of shame, and it gives you permission to keep showing up even when you don't feel like it.

That means your goals need to be *flexible*, not fragile. If they fall apart the second you hit a rough week, they're not strong enough.

They need to be *action-based*, not outcome-obsessed. You can't control your A1C every week, but you *can* choose to check your numbers, move your body, or drink your water.

And they need to be kind, instead of punishing. This isn't about earning rest or food or worthiness. It's about support.

When you create goals rooted in compassion instead of control, you give yourself a plan you can actually live with.

We've been brainwashed to think that if something feels easy, it's not enough.

But the truth is, your brain thrives on small wins. Every time you keep a promise to yourself, no matter how small, you build confidence and start rebuilding self-trust. You prove to yourself that you *can* follow through.

That's the foundation of consistency and the stuff that lasts longer than a streak of "perfect days."

The goal isn't to be impressive, but to be consistent enough that you don't have to keep starting over.

So instead of "I'll change everything on Monday," try this:

"I'll add one thing this week that makes life a little easier."

Because if your goals can't survive your bad days, they don't deserve your good ones.

And listen, it's important to remember, every big plan has a middle. You know, the part where excitement fades but results haven't shown up yet. That's where most people quit because the middle is uncomfortable, uncertain, and it's not sexy.

But that's where real change happens.

If you can stay in the process long enough to see the boring parts through, you'll realize that consistency doesn't require constant motivation. It requires your refusal to disappear.

———

What Helped Me Most

What helped me most was redefining what it means to "stick with it."

I used to think consistency meant perfection. I'd set the expectation of never missing a workout, never falling off track, and never needing to rest. But that wasn't motivation, it was me trying to control everything.

Now, I treat consistency like a heartbeat. It's steady, forgiving, sometimes fast, sometimes slow, but always present.

I stopped setting goals that demanded perfection and started setting *enough goals*.

Goals that fit my energy, my time, and my reality, and goals that could stay flexible when I felt like I couldn't.

When I miss a day, I don't start over, I just continue.

Because I'm not restarting. I'm returning.

My "bare minimum" goals are simple:

Drink the water.

Move a little.

Check my blood sugar once.

That's it. And that's enough.

And those small acts built more progress and more peace than any all-or-nothing plan ever did.

So if you're tired of setting goals that make you feel like you're constantly failing, here's your green light:

Shrink them.

Soften them.

Make them realistic.

Because the goal is consistent participation, not perfection.

And showing up, even halfway, still moves you forward.

That's what goal setting that doesn't suck looks like.

Mary Van Doorn

———

the power of one thing

. . .

“Small disciplines repeated with consistency every day lead to great achievements gained slowly over time.”

— John C. Maxwell

LET'S start with a truth bomb: all-or-nothing thinking is a trap and consistency has nothing to do with perfection.

If you've been living with type 2 diabetes for a while, you already know the cycle. You get motivated, maybe after a tough doctor's appointment or a scary number on your meter, and you decide: *This is it. This time I'm all in.* You clean out the pantry, swear off sugar, buy the journal, the supplements, the workout shoes, and maybe even a fancy blender that promises to change your life.

And for a few days, it works. You feel unstoppable, like you've finally cracked the code.

Until…life.

In comes a stressful week, a skipped workout, or a high blood sugar reading you can't explain. And just like that, the little voice creeps in:

You blew it. Might as well start over Monday.

That's the trap. We've been taught that success has to be extreme to count and that one detour means we've lost our way completely.

But real change? It doesn't happen in the extremes.

It happens in the middle, on the days when you're tired, distracted, cranky, and still manage to do *one thing* that keeps you tethered to your goals.

Been There, Felt That

"I used to think I had to do everything perfectly for it to count. If I didn't start on a Monday with a full grocery haul, a color-coded calendar, and zero slip-ups, I'd already failed. Turns out, one small shift, done consistently, did more for my progress than any perfect plan ever did."

The Magic of One Thing

The power of *one thing* is that it always fits.

One glass of water when you'd rather grab a soda.

One 10-minute walk when the gym feels impossible.

One moment to breathe before you react to a frustrating number on your CGM.

One pause to ask, *Am I hungry or just overwhelmed?*

One thing, done often, builds a foundation that no "perfect week" can match.

When you stop waiting to do everything "right," you finally create space to do something real. And that's where momentum lives. It's not in grand gestures, but in the quiet rhythm of showing up again and again.

Over time, one thing becomes two. A glass of water becomes a whole hydration habit, and a walk after dinner becomes a movement routine you actually enjoy. Checking your blood sugar without shame becomes data you can work with instead of dread you avoid.

That's how change happens. It grows quietly, one act of care at a time.

Why This Works (Even When It Feels Too Simple)

We love big promises because they feel powerful. Big goals look impressive. They make us feel like we're in control. But big goals also come with big pressure and pressure is fragile.

Small steps can survive the chaos. They meet you where you are instead of waiting for "someday," and they help you rebuild trust with yourself.

Each time you follow through, on the small, doable stuff, you send your brain a message: *I can count on me.*

That's how confidence is built. Not from hype or perfect streaks, but from gentle, consistent proof that you'll keep showing up.

The "one thing" approach also keeps your nervous system out of fight-or-flight mode. You're no longer trying to sprint your way to peace. You're walking toward it slowly, intentionally, and sustainably.

And here's the best part: one thing doesn't just fit into your life, it also *adapts* to it.

Bad day? One thing.

Busy week? One thing.

Burnout creeping in? Still, one thing.

You're never starting from zero again, because you always have something that anchors you.

The Real-Life Version of This

I know this sounds simple, but simple doesn't mean easy.

Some days your "one thing" might be just checking your blood sugar once instead of avoiding it.

Other days, it might be going for a walk even though you'd rather scroll your phone.

And sometimes, it might be saying, "I'm going to bed early because everything else can wait."

That's strategy, not slacking.

The world loves to celebrate extremes. It celebrates crash diets, miracle programs, and overnight transformations, but none of those things teach you how to live. *One thing* does.

One thing is how you stay in motion without burning out, stay kind to yourself while still making progress, and how you stop the quit restart cycle, and start living.

This isn't about being basic. It's about being brilliantly consistent.

We've been trained to chase motivation and wait for perfect timing, but motivation is flaky and perfection is fake. And timing? Never going to be perfect.

Consistency is where your power lives. It's the quiet determination to keep showing up, even when no one notices.

So stop measuring your success by how many things you can juggle and start measuring it by how many times you chose one small thing. And then, kept choosing it.

That's how health gets built.

Not in the all or nothing.

In the *showing up anyway*.

———

What Helped Me Most

For years, I thought progress had to feel like a sprint. I'd plan every detail, wait for the right moment, and throw myself into change with wild enthusiasm only to burn out by week three. I was doing everything and nothing at the same time.

What helped me most was realizing that real success feels slower, quieter, and gentler.

It was learning that I didn't need to "start over" every time life knocked me sideways. I just needed to return to my *one thing*.

Some days that meant lacing up my shoes for a gentle walk.

Other days, it meant drinking one glass of water and calling it a win.

And sometimes, it just meant taking a deep breath and choosing not to spiral.

Over time, that consistency created something I'd been chasing for years: peace.

I finally stopped treating my health like a project and started treating it like a partnership, and I began to trust myself again.

And that trust, built one small act at a time, became the most powerful part of my journey.

So if you're staring at another "fresh start," ready to overhaul everything, I want you to pause.

You don't need to fix your whole life.

You just need to pick your one thing.

Because one thing, done with heart, done again tomorrow and the next day and the next, is enough to change everything.

———

movement that
works for you

. . .

"Exercise should be a celebration of what your body can do, not a punishment for what you ate."

— Unknown

FOR A LOT OF US, the word *exercise* came wrapped in shame.

It wasn't something we did out of joy, only something we did out of guilt. We were taught that moving our bodies was the price we paid for what we ate. That "working out" was what disciplined people did while the rest of us needed to "try harder."

For years, movement felt like punishment disguised as self-care. It was gym class humiliation, diet challenges, and "no pain, no gain" slogans yelled by people who had no idea what our lives were really like.

No wonder so many of us have side-eyed the treadmill for years.

But here's the truth no one told us when we were hustling through burpees we hated and pretending not to feel embarrassed in group classes:

Your body doesn't need punishment. It needs partnership.

Movement is not a penance. It's a gift . Think of it as a daily chance to feel more alive, more grounded, and more *you*.

Been There, Felt That

"I used to move my body out of guilt, like I owed it something for every bite I took. Every workout felt like a punishment or a payback. But once I stopped tying movement to food and started noticing how it helped my mood, my stress, and my energy, my attitude toward movement softened. Now I move because it supports me, and not because I'm trying to earn anything."

Redefining What Counts

At some point, we absorbed the idea that movement only counts if it looks hard, is sweat-drenched, timed, tracked, or performed in a gym full of mirrors.

But your body doesn't care if you're doing squats in fancy leggings or dancing in your kitchen in pajama pants. It just wants to move.

A ten-minute walk after dinner, stretching while watching TV, boxing in VR, vacuuming your living room, or playing tag with your grandkids. It all counts.

Movement doesn't have to be structured or epic to be effective. It just has to exist.

Your body keeps score of all the small things, not just the Instagram-worthy ones.

What Movement Can Be (When It's Not Punishment)

When you take shame out of the equation, movement stops being a chore and starts being a conversation.

Some days, it's a mood reset, a way to shake off frustration or anxiety.

Other days, it's a way to stabilize blood sugar or clear mental fog.

Sometimes, it's quiet, gentle stretches that remind you you're still here, and still capable.

Sometimes, it's playful…dancing, swimming, or walking with music blasting in your ears.

Movement can be self-respect instead of self-correction.

It's not about shrinking your body, but about supporting it.

And it's not about controlling yourself, but about connecting to yourself.

When you move for how it *feels*, not how it *looks*, you start to experience the real payoff: energy, strength, stress relief, confidence, and the sweet realization that your body has been on your side all along.

Finding Your Fit (Literally and Figuratively)

You're allowed to like the way you move. Radical right?

You're allowed to choose joy over grind.

If the gym feels like a chore but nature fills your cup, take the walk.

If yoga calms your nerves more than cardio ever did, roll out the mat.

If strength training makes you feel powerful, awesome. Do that.

If VR workouts, dance breaks, or stretching on the floor bring you peace, you do you boo.

Movement isn't one-size-fits-all. It's personal. It should fit your season of life, your energy level, and your reality, not someone else's version of "discipline."

If you haven't found your "thing" yet, that doesn't mean you hate exercise. It probably means you've only been introduced to the versions that made you feel smaller, instead of stronger.

When Motivation Disappears (Because It Will)

Let's just call it what it is. Some days you're a whole motivational poster, and some days the couch is your soulmate. Totally normal.

That's because motivation is a spark, not fuel.

The key is having gentle entry points that keep you in motion even when you don't "feel like it."

Maybe it's a single song you dance to while cooking dinner or marching in place while your coffee brews. It could be parking farther away from the store to sneak in a few extra steps, or one deep stretch before bed to show your body a little love.

Those little movements compound, and they shift your mood. Not only do they wake up your circulation, but they also wake up your confidence, and your *self-trust*.

Because the goal isn't perfection, it's participation. And sometimes participation looks like walking to the mailbox and calling it enough for today.

The Emotional Side of Movement

For many of us, rebuilding a healthy relationship with movement also means grieving the years we spent hating it, or hating ourselves through it.

We have to let go of the idea that exercise is a moral test you either pass or fail.

It also means forgiving yourself for the seasons you stopped moving because it was too painful, either physically or emotionally, or both.

It means realizing that rest counts too and that choosing gentleness for yourself over punishment is still progress.

When you start seeing movement as something that helps your life and not something that bosses you around, it gets a whole lot easier to show up. The dread fades, because it's no longer something you use to beat yourself up.

———

What Helped Me Most

For years, I measured the success of my workouts by sweat, soreness, and calories burned. If I missed a day, I felt lazy. If I couldn't push hard, I felt weak. If I didn't see results fast enough, I assumed it wasn't working.

What helped me most was redefining movement as *medicine, not punishment.*

When I started moving in ways that felt good instead of forced, my relationship with exercise changed.

I walked to clear my head instead of to "earn dinner."

I danced to shift my energy instead of to shrink my body.

I stretched to reconnect with myself instead of to check off a box.

And I stopped asking, "Is this enough?" and started asking, "Does this support me today?"

That mindset freed me from the guilt that had kept me stuck. Ten minutes stopped feeling like a failure and started feeling like a promise kept to myself.

Now, movement is something I do *for* me, not *to* me.

Some days it's sweaty and some days it's slow, but it all still counts.

So if you've been avoiding exercise because it feels like a chore, or because you're scared of doing it wrong, this is your sign:

Start where you are. Do what you can. And let it feel good.

You don't have to punish yourself to make progress.

You just have to move. Your way, at your pace, following your own rules.

The best movement plan isn't the hardest one, it's the one that keeps you coming back.

And that's the movement that works for you.

———

redefining wellness (and what self-care actually means)

. . .

"Self-care is not a luxury—it's a radical act of self-preservation."

— Audre Lorde

WELLNESS ISN'T A PRODUCT, a cleanse, or a hashtag.

It's not a fancy supplement routine, a color-coordinated gym outfit, or a $75 candle named *Serenity Now*. It's not lemon water at sunrise, a silent yoga retreat, or a perfectly filtered morning routine that starts at 5 a.m. and somehow includes journaling, meditation, and a side of enlightenment.

Somewhere along the way, self-care got hijacked by hustle culture and it stopped being about feeling better and started being about *looking* like you had it all together. Now it's less "take care of yourself" and more "perform your wellness for the internet."

And honestly? That performative version is exhausting, expensive, and totally unrealistic. Especially when you're managing a chronic condition like type 2 diabetes and when your days already revolve around energy crashes, meal timing, meds, appointments, and trying to stay functional, instead of flawless.

So let's take it back. Let's talk about what *real* wellness looks like.

Been There, Felt That

"I used to think self-care was supposed to feel soft and luxurious like candles, baths, and all the pretty things. But real self-care? Sometimes it's checking my blood sugar when I don't want to, ordering refills before I run out, or canceling plans because my body is asking for rest. It's not glamorous, but it's the stuff that actually keeps me going."

What Wellness Isn't

For years, I thought wellness was a checklist, like a series of gold stars I could earn if I just did enough.

If I worked out enough, ate clean enough, or meditated enough, maybe then I'd *deserve* rest.

But wellness isn't a competition or a punishment, and it's not a perfectly executed routine that makes you worthy of approval.

And it's definitely not something you earn by suffering first.

True wellness doesn't need to impress anyone. It doesn't require a rigid schedule, a "clean" label, or a constant performance of positivity.

Wellness isn't about proving you have control over your life. It's about building a life that supports you even when you don't.

What Real Self-Care Looks Like

Real self-care is rarely fancy. Most of the time, it's maintenance. The small, quiet choices that keep your life livable and your body supported.

It looks like saying no, even when guilt shows up loud and uninvited. Taking your medication without the internal eye roll. Letting yourself rest when your body taps out, even if the dishes are still sitting there judging you. It's walking into a doctor's appointment with questions instead of nodding along and hoping for the best. It's choosing something simple to eat rather than skipping meals and calling it discipline.

Self-care can be going to bed early, taking a walk without tracking every step, or ignoring texts for a night because your brain is done.

It can also be the unglamorous stuff. Calling the pharmacy again. Pushing back on insurance. Setting boundaries that make other people uncomfortable but keep you intact.

It doesn't have to be cute.

It just has to help you.

The "I'm Too Tired" Truth

If you've ever said, "I know what to do, I'm just too tired to do it," know this: you're not lazy or unmotivated. You're *tired*.

I'm talking about the kind of tired that seeps into your bones. The physical fatigue mixed with mental load, decision fatigue, emotional burnout, and blood-sugar swings that make your body feel like it's constantly buffering.

Recognizing this kind of exhaustion is eye-opening data.

When your body and mind are both running on fumes, even simple tasks start to feel impossible. Real wellness doesn't ask you to bulldoze that burnout, just to notice it.

It asks you to trade perfection for compassion, to shift the question from *"What's the absolute healthiest thing I could do right now?"* to *"What would feel nourishing right now?"*

Some days nourishment is a salad and a walk.

Other days it's meds, water, and a solid nap.

Both count and both are self-care.

You Don't Owe Anyone a Vibe

You don't have to look like you have your life together to be taking care of yourself.

You don't owe the world an aesthetic. You don't need curated meals or perfect gym selfies, or to prove your worth through your wellness routine.

Your wellness doesn't have to be pretty to be powerful.

Sometimes it's a walk outside to clear your head, or stretching on the couch between meetings.

Sometimes it's silence instead of screens, and sometimes it's sitting with your emotions instead of eating or scrolling them away.

The most radical act of self-care is tuning in instead of tuning out.

———

What Helped Me Most

What helped me most was realizing that self-care isn't something I have to *earn*, but something I'm allowed to *need*.

For years, I treated rest as a reward and wellness as a report card.

If I was "good," I could relax. If I was "bad," I had to double down.

But all that did was keep me trapped in a loop of striving and shame.

Eventually, I started asking a different question:

What does support look like right now?

Sometimes that meant practical support like refilling a prescription, prepping a meal I'll actually eat, or scheduling a follow-up before it becomes a crisis.

Sometimes it meant emotional support like allowing myself to cry, saying no without an explanation, or admitting I was overwhelmed.

And sometimes it meant spiritual support: stepping back, breathing, and reminding myself that I'm not a machine.

Real self-care didn't always feel indulgent or pretty. Often times it was messy, uncomfortable, or unglamorous. But it made my life *work*.

Now, I don't chase a vibe. I protect my peace, support my body, and choose actions that make me feel aligned, not admired.

Because wellness isn't about being perfect.

It's about being *present*.

And self-care? It's how you keep showing up for your life, even when it's hard, chaotic, and beautifully imperfect.

—

celebrating progress, not just results

. . .

"Don't wait until you reach your goal to be proud of yourself. Be proud of every step you take toward it."

— Karen Salmansohn

TRUTH BOMB:

You're allowed to be proud of yourself even if nothing "spectacular" happened this week.

No gold stars.

No side-by-side photos.

No shiny numbers on a scale.

Just you, showing up, choosing yourself, and living the work.

That's what matters, and that's where the real progress lives.

Been There, Felt That

"I didn't lose a pound this month, but I checked my blood sugar every day, showed up for my workouts, and didn't skip my meds once. That used to be 'failing.' Now I call it growth."

. . .

The Problem with "Before and After"

We live in a world obsessed with transformation stories.

The big reveal, the jaw-dropping side-by-side, and the moment that makes everyone say, "Wow, I didn't even recognize you."

And sure, those stories can be inspiring, but they can also be misleading. Because the truth is, the "after" photo is just a snapshot in time. It doesn't show the late-night doubts, the skipped workouts, or the days you wanted to quit but didn't.

When the spotlight stays on *results*, we start believing that progress only counts when it's visible and that if our changes don't look impressive, they must not be real or worth of celebration.

But that's a lie.

The most meaningful progress often happens quietly in the moments no one claps for, and in the habits no one sees.

The progress that changes you the most rarely fits in a "before and after."

What Real Progress Actually Looks Like

Progress isn't flashy. It's the small choices you make when no one's watching. It's checking your blood sugar even when you're nervous about the number, or cooking at home when it would be easier to swing through the drive thru.

Progress is taking your meds when you'd rather pretend you don't need them, pausing before stress-eating and asking yourself what you really need. It's choosing rest without guilt. It's walking around the block because you promised yourself you would.

Those moments may not get likes or applause, but they matter so much more than you think.

Because they're evidence of growth, instead of perfection.

They're proof that you're learning to care for yourself on purpose and you are becoming the kind of person who shows up, even when the outcome isn't guaranteed.

And that? It's everything when it comes to your wellness.

. . .

The Mindset That Holds Us Back

So many of us downplay our wins with a single phrase: *"Yeah, but..."*

Yeah, but I still have a long way to go.

Yeah, but I missed two workouts last week.

Yeah, but my A1C hasn't budged yet.

We talk ourselves out of pride because we've been trained to believe only perfection deserves celebration. But that mindset is what keeps you stuck in a cycle of disappointment.

You don't have to *earn* pride and you don't have to cross a finish line before you're allowed to clap for yourself.

You are living inside a body that sometimes fights you, and still, you show up. You keep trying and caring. That's not a small thing. It's strength in motion.

So the next time your brain tries to minimize a win, interrupt it.

Replace *"yeah, but..."* with *"actually, yeah."*

Actually, yeah, I walked today.

Actually, yeah, I took my meds.

Actually, yeah, I checked in with myself instead of ignoring how I felt.

And actually, yeah, that totally counts.

Why Celebrating Progress Matters

Celebration isn't fluff, it's fuel.

Your brain is wired to repeat what it's rewarded for. When you acknowledge your efforts, you reinforce them, and you remind yourself: *I can do this.*

When you only celebrate the big stuff, you starve your motivation. But when you celebrate the daily work, the "boring" stuff, you start to build momentum.

And momentum is what gets you through the weeks that feel heavy, and what reminds you that you're not starting from scratch, even when you're struggling.

Progress and confidence both compound.

And so does self-trust, every time you give yourself credit where it's due.

————

What Helped Me Most

For most of my life, I only celebrated outcomes.

If the number didn't go down, if the chart didn't improve, if my jeans didn't fit differently, I decided I had failed.

I was working hard, but I never felt accomplished. I was doing better, but I couldn't see it.

And that mindset kept me in a constant loop of frustration.

What helped me most was changing what I measured.

I stopped waiting for visible progress to validate my effort and I started celebrating the invisible stuff.

The morning I checked my blood sugar instead of avoiding it.

The night I went to bed early instead of scrolling until midnight.

The moment I caught a spiral and said, "Nope, not today."

The walk I took when I didn't feel like moving at all.

The boundary I set when people-pleasing would've been easier.

None of those things earned me a medal, but they earned me momentum.

And that momentum turned into confidence, the quiet kind that builds over time, and the kind that doesn't need a transformation photo to prove it's real.

Now, I celebrate everything. Every step, every effort, and every choice that moves me closer to the life I want.

Because every time I say, *"That counted,"* I'm rewriting the story of who I am.

I'm not waiting to feel proud, I'm practicing it.

I'm not waiting for perfect, I'm building consistency.

And I'm not waiting for applause, I'm giving it to my damn self.

So the next time you're tempted to shrug off your effort with a "yeah, but…," stop yourself.

Take a breath.

Smile.
And say it instead:
"Actually, yeah. I did that. And it's awesome."
Because it is.
And so are you.

———

wrapping up part 3: habits, healing, and everyday wins

"You don't have to move mountains to change your life.
Sometimes you just have to keep showing up."

— Unknown

This is where it all comes together.

The awareness, the mindset shifts, and the small, steady steps that add up over time.

This part was never about overhauling your life, but about learning to live it differently.

On your terms. At your pace. With compassion leading the way.

Because healing, real healing, doesn't happen in a single breakthrough moment.

It happens in the daily choices that don't always look spectacular but feel solid.

It's in the water you drink when you'd rather have soda.

The walk you take when your motivation's missing.

The quiet "no" you give when you need rest more than people-pleasing.

It's the trust you build every time you show up, even imperfectly.

You've unlearned so much: diet culture, perfectionism, comparison, and shame. And you've replaced it with something stronger-self-respect.

You've learned that wellness isn't about control. It's about connection.

And that discipline means nothing without compassion.

Most importantly you've learned health isn't a finish line, it's a relationship.

What Helped Me Most

What helped me most was finally understanding that consistency and compassion can coexist.

I used to think I had to choose between going all in or giving up.

But it turns out, I just needed to keep going, with grace in the passenger seat.

I stopped waiting for motivation and started relying more on momentum.

I stopped measuring progress by what anyone else could see and started measuring it by how I felt.

I started celebrating the days I followed through, yes, but also the days I simply refused to quit on myself.

That's what healing looks like now. It's not perfect days, but steady ones. Not performing wellness, but actually living it.

So here's the truth I hope you carry with you:

You don't need a new version of yourself, you just need to keep honoring the one you're becoming.

You've done the hard work of showing up for your mind, your body, and your life in a way that's real, sustainable, and yours.

This isn't about "getting back on track."

You *are* the track.

Keep trusting your body, protecting your peace, and celebrating the progress no one else can see.

Because this grounded, imperfect, intentional version of you
is exactly where the healing lives.

Wrapping Up Part 3: Habits, Healing, and Everyday Wins

the final chapter: this isn't the end-it's a reboot

"You don't have to have it all figured out to keep moving forward."

— Morgan Harper Nichols

Let's get one thing straight:

This is not the end of your story.

You didn't read your way to perfection.

You didn't arrive at a magical destination where motivation never fades and carbs always cooperate.

And you're not supposed to.

Because managing type 2 diabetes, hell, *managing life*, isn't about mastering every moment.

It's about showing up anyway.

It's about learning to keep going after the messy days, the high numbers, the missed workouts, the nights you cry in your car and eat snacks in bed.

You don't need a reset button.

You need rhythm.

You need realness.

You need a *reboot*...because you're evolving, not because you've failed.

So, What Did We Learn?

Let's break it down. If nothing else sticks, let *this* sink in:

🩸 **You are not your numbers.**

Your A1C is not your worth. Your blood sugar is not your moral compass. Data is just information. It's not a report card.

🧠 **Mindset is medicine.**

The thoughts you believe shape your health more than any rulebook ever will. You don't need toxic positivity. You need honest belief in yourself.

💬 **Stigma is a liar.**

You didn't do this to yourself. You're not "bad" for needing meds. You are not broken. You are navigating something real, and you deserve support.

🏃 **Action beats motivation.**

You won't always *feel* like doing the thing. Do it anyway. Tiny steps, boring steps, Tuesday afternoon steps. They all count.

🧂 **Balance > willpower.**

Perfection isn't sustainable. Progress is. You can live well and still eat a cookie. You can be healthy and still rest.

💥 **Quitting isn't failure.**

It's data. If something isn't working, it's not you, it's the strategy. Adjust, don't abandon.

🤝 **Support matters.**

You weren't meant to do this alone. Whether it's one friend, a coach, or a whole community. Find your people. Let them hold you up.

🩶 **You can be a work in progress and still be worthy.**

You don't need to arrive to deserve peace. You don't need to shrink to be celebrated. You are allowed to love yourself *while* you grow.

————

What Helped Me Most

What helped me most was learning to stop waiting for a clean slate.

For years, I thought progress meant starting over every Monday, every first-of-the-month, or every January.

I thought if I could just "do it right," I'd finally become someone who had it all together.

But that mindset kept me in a loop of all-or-nothing, shame, and disappointment.

What finally set me free?

Letting it be messy. Letting it be mine. And letting it be enough.

I stopped saying, "I'll try again when things calm down."

I started asking, "What's one thing I can do today, even in the crazy?"

I learned to look at my blood sugar without spiraling.

To take my meds without guilt.

To move my body without punishing it.

To forgive myself *without* starting over.

And the wildest part?

That's when the real progress started.

Because when you stop quitting on yourself, your life changes.

————

Keep Going, But Make It Yours

You don't have to hustle your way into health.

You don't need to white-knuckle your way to worthiness.

You don't have to look like anyone else's before-and-after.

You get to do this *differently now*.

You get to take care of yourself *without* shame.

You get to rewrite the narrative you've been sold about diabetes.

You get to live fully, not in spite of your diagnosis, but *alongside it*.

You didn't choose this path.

But you're here. You're showing up. You're learning.

And that? That's badass.

This isn't a "goodbye." It's a "you got this."

It's a "see you out there."

It's a "DM me when you eat something amazing and don't feel bad about it."

The book may end here. But your story doesn't.

And I can't wait to see how you write the next chapter.

a note to you, the reader

Hey, you.

Yeah, *you*-the one who just made it through this entire book.

First of all: I'm proud of you.

Not just for reading every chapter, but for showing up for yourself. For being open to doing this differently. For making space to think, reflect, and maybe even laugh a little while tackling something as heavy (and frustrating and real) as living with type 2 diabetes.

If this book felt like a conversation with a friend, that was the goal. Because we need less shame, more support. Less diet dogma, more truth. Fewer rules, and more real talk.

And I'm not going anywhere.

If you want more support, resources, or just someone who *gets it*, come hang out with me online. I post mindset tips, diabetes truths, and the occasional meme that says what we're all thinking.

Come say hi:

 Instagram: @sms_diabetes_support

 Facebook: Sugar Mama Strong Diabetes Support
Dudes with Diabetes-Diabetes Support for Men

 Podcast: *Sick of Pricks* -Real talk for real life with type 2

🌐 Or check out www.sugarmamastrong.com for updates, resources, and all the things.

And if this book spoke to you, I'd be honored if you shared it with a friend, a fellow warrior, or even your doctor. Because the more we talk about type 2 diabetes with honesty and humanity, the more we break the cycle of stigma.

Thanks for letting me be a small part of your journey. I'm cheering you on every step of the way.

With love,
Mary
Your diabetes bestie 💕

about the author

Mary Van Doorn is the founder of Sugar Mama Strong, a thriving community for people living with diabetes who want support, accountability, and real conversations about health. After her own diagnosis and years of navigating shame, confusion, and burnout, she built the resources and community she wished she had from the start. Through coaching, education, and unfiltered storytelling, Mary has helped thousands of people feel seen, supported, and capable of creating a life that feels good again.

www.ingramcontent.com/pod-product-compliance
Lightning Source LLC
Chambersburg PA
CBHW022205050726
47590CB00002B/653